Chaos and Organization in Health Care

Chaos and Organization in Health Care

Thomas H. Lee, MD, and James J. Mongan, MD

The MIT Press
Cambridge, Massachusetts
London, England

For information about special discounts, please email
<special_sales@mitpress.mit.edu>.

This book was set in Palatino by SNP Best-set Typesetter Ltd., Hong Kong.
Printed and bound in the United States of America.

Library of Congress Cataloging-in-Publication Data

Lee, Thomas H.
Chaos and organization in health care / Thomas H. Lee, M.D. and James J. Mongan, M.D.
    p. cm.
Includes bibliographical references and index.
ISBN 978-0-262-01353-6 (hardcover : alk. paper) 1. Medical care—United States. 2. Health care reform—United States. 3. Health facilities—United States—Administration. 4. Chaotic behavior in systems. 5. Organizational behavior. I. Mongan, James J. II. Title.
RA395.A3L414   2009
362.1′04250973—dc22

2009013164

10 9 8 7 6 5 4 3 2 1

To our families:
Soheyla, Simin, Sabrina, and Ariana,
and
Jean, Sarah, John, and Theresa

Contents

Introduction

As daunting as the challenges for U.S. health care may be, there is reason for optimism that a delivery system that is much more efficient, reliable, and safe is within our reach. Our optimism is derived not from theory but from our day-to-day work, which ranges from health policy leadership roles to the management of an academic integrated delivery system to hands-on patient care. From this work, we have a frontline view of the good that modern medicine can produce, but also the inefficiency, missed opportunities, confusion, and occasional harm. We see the consequences of a lack of health insurance for individual patients and understand the challenges of making coverage for all work.

Despite the magnitude and diversity of these challenges, we are optimistic because we believe that they share a common "root cause"—and that this root cause is vulnerable to attack. We in fact see signs of real progress in provider organizations around the country, including our own. Simply put, our assessment is:

- The problem is chaos
- The solution is organization
- The question is how we get there

The Problem Is Chaos

It would be good news if rising health care costs could be explained by the greed of specific individuals or companies, because then those individuals and companies could be stopped. And it would be good news if disappointing quality and lapses in safety could be blamed on the incompetence of specific physicians, because then those doctors could undergo more training or their licenses could be revoked. "Bad guys" who are greedy or incompetent do exist in medicine, of course, but the unfortunate news is that these bad guys play relatively small roles in the creation of our crises in health care.

Indeed, the big driver of our problems is an undisputed "good guy"—progress itself, which when imposed on the fragmented U.S. health care system, produces chaos. Let us explain what we mean by progress, fragmentation, and chaos.

We are lucky to live in an era during which medical science is racing ahead, producing advances that are easily taken for granted—that is, unless you are a patient or doctor. During our careers, we have seen incurable diseases become routinely curable—like the lymphoma that was diagnosed in September 2006 in Red Sox pitcher John Lester, but eradicated in time for him to join spring training in 2007 and pitch a no-hitter in 2008. Fatal diseases like HIV have become controllable chronic conditions with a surprisingly modest impact on life expectancy. And common diseases have become preventable—like heart attacks, the death toll from which has steadily declined because of the widespread use of medications that control blood pressure and cholesterol.

We are not among those who wax nostalgic for the simpler and less costly health care of a generation ago. To be a doctor today is to know there is virtually always *something* you can do for a patient, no matter how sick he or she might be. We like that.

But to be a doctor today—or a patient—is to be overwhelmed by an explosion of new knowledge. That explosion produces multiple options for testing and treating conditions for which there were none just a few years ago. The knowledge explosion also means that giving complex patients state-of-the-art care requires multiple physicians with highly specialized expertise. These physicians need to communicate with each other, and ideally, should develop clear game plans with patients and their families.

Unfortunately, this explosion of knowledge has gone off within a health care delivery system that is poorly prepared to help physicians make the best decisions or work effectively together. Most office visits in the United States are at small practices with one or two doctors, who write prescriptions on prescription pads and store notes in paper charts. These doctors work hard, but they work in isolation, struggling to stay up to date on the best ways to help their patients. Many settle for a more modest goal: just staying one step in front of their patients, who often bring printouts from the Internet to office visits.

An even greater challenge for these isolated physicians is providing *coordinated* care for their patients—a goal that requires knowing what other doctors are doing and saying. A generation ago, these physicians might have seen each other in the hospital, and discussed their shared patients in hallways, lunchrooms, or doctors' lounges. But today there are many more doctors involved in the care of complex patients, and these doctors are frequently in different institutions. And the pace of medical life has accelerated so that these conversations occur less reliably or not at all. The doctors' dining rooms and lounges have disappeared, because no one has time to sit in them anymore.

The result is chaos. There is too much to do and not enough time to do it. There are too many people involved, and they are not actually talking to each other. There are plenty of good intentions and a lot of hard work—but there is also duplication of efforts, dropped balls, mixed messages, and poor coordination.

Patients have to answer the same questions over and over, and still wonder if their providers remember who they are. These patients find themselves confused about issues so basic that they are often embarrassed to seek clarification by asking questions such as "Who is in charge?" "What am I supposed to do next?" and "What medications should I be taking?"

The Solution Is Organization

We believe that the best way to address health care's cost and quality crises is to attack this chaos. Health care spending will inevitably rise as people live longer and breakthroughs occur, but increases can be mitigated if clinicians have help identifying the best strategies for evaluating and treating patients, and if they work in teams that help patients avoid hospitalizations and stay as healthy as possible. These teams should include physicians, nurses, pharmacists, and social workers—as well as patients themselves.

Yet teams need structure, leadership, communication tools, and "playbooks" that are understood by all involved. In short, they need organization, so that patients and their clinicians can work together efficiently and effectively.

We believe that the organization of health care should be a clear and unifying goal in discussions of how health care should be financed, and the roles of consumerism and other market forces. The afflictions of modern medicine—high costs and disappointing quality—exist in every developed country, which suggests that the method of financing health care is unlikely to provide a solution on its own. And while we have a healthy respect for the potential influence of market forces in health care, we believe that their greatest impact comes from rewarding the performance that can only be accomplished through more organized care.

The concept of organized health care is not an abstract ideal. Around the United States, well-organized health care providers like the Mayo Clinic, Virginia Mason Medical Center in Seattle, Washington, and Geisinger Health System in Danville, Pennsylvania, are adapting management principles from non-health care industries. They strive to become "high-reliability organizations," and use words like "guarantees" and "promises" to describe their care. Compared to the fragmented mainstream of U.S. health care, these organizations deliver care that is by many measures safer, of a higher quality, and less costly. These "tight" organizations are unusual in that their physicians are generally salaried employees of the parent company. But other organizations (including our own) are watching and learning, and are adapting their approaches for academic medical centers and providers in the community.

A patient who is seeing a physician doesn't really care whether that physician is a salaried employee or a partner in a group practice. What matters to the patient is the quality of the doctor's care. Thus, the organizational structure of providers is most important as the context for implementation of a range of systems that lead to the actual improvements in care, including:

• Information systems, such as electronic medical records, that help physicians make better decisions as individuals (e.g., prescribing the most cost-effective drugs) and work well in teams—because their colleagues can see what they have done.

• Team-based care, which allows practices to meet patients' needs outside of doctor visits. One example is the use of registries to keep track of patients with diabetes, enabling a diabetes educator to contact patients who may not have come in for recent office visits.

• Disease management programs to improve the coordination of care of the sickest and most complex patients—an important approach both to improve quality and control costs, since just 5 percent of patients account for about 50 percent of health care spending.

The potential of these and other systems to improve efficiency and quality is real, but most health care providers have been too fragmented to develop such programs—or even to sign the types of contracts with health plans that would reward providers for doing so. Accordingly, health plans have stepped into the void and done what they could to supply organization to health care. In chapter 8, we describe the contributions made by health plans as well as employers and patients toward improving care through greater organization. We think these efforts are important and valuable, but their impact can be considerably enhanced if combined with organized providers who use systems to improve care.

How Do We Get There?

Our descriptions of organized health care in the second section of this book may be unfamiliar to many readers, but we doubt that its potential value will be controversial. The difficult question is, How do we get there? What policy, market, and cultural changes will accelerate the development of a better-organized, higher-performing health care system?

Our "prescription" is explained in the third section of this book. There is, of course, no single magic bullet. Instead, we believe that multiple strategies should be used with the common goal of encouraging health care providers to become participants in effective delivery organizations, and then encourage those organizations to achieve higher and higher performance.

In an ideal world and a perfectly rational health care marketplace, all Americans might get their health care within tightly structured delivery organizations in which the providers are paid not for the volume of services delivered but rather for meeting the needs of their patient population. We don't live in such a world, however, and the spread of this ideal model has been limited by a medical culture in which physicians prize their autonomy and patients prize the option to seek care from whomever they choose—even if it is outside their "network" of providers. Tightly organized care is especially difficult to imagine in rural settings, where there are fewer providers, and they are separated by greater distances. Organized care can also be difficult to implement at academic medical centers, which attract patients with more complex illnesses, and in many cases, a strong interest in intense testing and treatment.

Despite these barriers, we should not give up on the goal of organizing U.S. health care to improve its performance. As depicted schematically in the figure below, we believe that the organizational stage of the evolution of providers (shown on x-axis) correlates with the payment methodologies that they can accommodate (y-axis). Physicians in solo practices are uncomfortable with any payment structure other than traditional fee-for-service. But at the other end of the spectrum, tightly structured organizations can assume complete clinical and financial responsibilities for a population's care under "capitation." Providers with intermediate organizational structures can accommodate payment methodologies with intermediate levels of risk.

For providers to move from the left to right, and for payment methods to move from the bottom to top, providers need to adopt the systems described on horizontal bars within the figure. Will such changes come

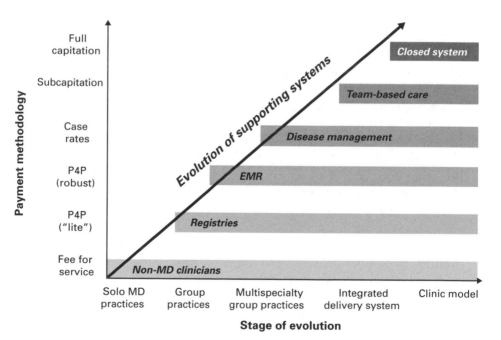

Figure I.1
Evolving reimbursement and care models. P4P = pay for performance; EMR = electronic medical records. (Reproduced with permission from TH Lee and RA Berenson, "The Organization of Health Care Delivery: A Roadmap for Accelerated Improvement," in *The Health Care Delivery System* [Washington, DC: Center for American Progress, 2008], available at <http://www.americanprogress.org/issues/2008/10/pdf/health_delivery_full.pdf>)

through gradual evolution? Or will they come through revolution—that is, abrupt and drastic change in the payment system? We believe there is a middle road, in which the organization of the provider world can be accelerated without the massive disruptions to care that would be inevitable with sudden major changes in payment methodology. In the third section of this book, we describe how progress of our health care marketplace toward the upper right corner of the figure can be accelerated through the thoughtful use of multiple strategies including public reporting, the flexible use of multiple payment models, and more than a little strong leadership from the provider community.

At its core, this is an optimistic book. In our youths, we were drawn to health care because we believed that medicine could improve the lives of patients. We remain confident in that belief today, and find ourselves similarly hopeful that the progress we see around the country and within our own organization signify that better health care is coming. That health care will be more efficient, more reliable, and safer, because clinicians are using systems that help them make the right decisions, and work more effectively with patients and each other.

How health care is financed is important. How market forces are activated is crucial. Yet we believe the influence of these approaches will be exerted through their ability to catalyze the organization of health care providers—in short, less chaos, more organization. Our hope is that this book will help shift the balance in the right direction.

I The Problem Is Chaos

1 Chaos

Her friends and doctors still describe her as "formidable," and at age eighty, SC finds that amusing. When she was younger and still teaching William Shakespeare to college students, she knew she was a force—a passionate, sometimes intimidating teacher who knew how to make her points. She used those same skills after she retired as a community activist—the sort of well-informed, overwhelmingly articulate citizen who just by walking into a public hearing, can cause local politicians' hearts to sink.

Today, she remains imposing. SC leans toward her listeners as she speaks, and they tend to lean ever so slightly backward. But the word *she* uses to describe herself is "vulnerable." She has a long list of medical problems, a cane, and many vials filled with pills. In the last few years, she has been diagnosed with three different cancers—chronic lymphocytic lymphoma, then skin cancer, and then lung cancer—and she suffers real aggravation every day from a long list of other conditions, including asthma, arthritis, heartburn, gout, high blood pressure, and hay fever.

As bad as those problems might be, SC is most troubled by the strange and scary spell in 2004 when she lost her memory. For several hours, she could walk, talk, and think—but she could not record new memories. People told her things, and the thought was instantly gone. She asked her partner the same questions over and over. And then, as mysteriously as it began, the spell was over.

At the time she thought she was having a stroke. Instead, after an extensive evaluation, she was told that she had transient global amnesia—more a description than a diagnosis, really, since transient global amnesia thus far has eluded scientific explanation. She has not had any recurrences, but she remains unnerved by the episode.

Over the years, SC has become accustomed to bad news about her lungs, joints, stomach, and blood cells, yet the idea that her *brain* might be vulnerable scares her. She has, after all, always felt that her mind is what defines her. Every day, she reads the *New York Times* and scours legal notices in the local paper for items relevant to her favored causes. But now she also uses the Internet to research her medications and diseases. When she finds something intriguing, she passes the information on to her doctors.

The work of communicating with those doctors—and trying to get them to communicate with each other—sometimes seems a full-time job. SC has a primary care physician and an allergist in the Rhode Island city where she lives. For most of her care, however, she drives fifty miles to Boston, where she sees an internist, an oncologist, a lung specialist, and an orthopedist. In 2006, she was admitted to the hospital for a total knee replacement, and in 2007, she had two procedures to diagnose and remove her lung cancer, and a third for a bladder problem. She had a total of eighteen Boston office visits with twelve different doctors (including one of the authors of this book) in 2007 alone. During that year, she underwent CT scans of her abdomen, chest, and pelvis—twice for each test. She also had her mammogram and a flu shot.

SC takes a *lot* of medications. Her eighteen active prescriptions overflowed her medicine cabinet long ago and now also fill the drawer in the nightstand by her bed. She gets chemotherapy for her lymphoma, and takes six medications for her asthma and an annoying cough. She uses other drugs for her arthritis, heartburn, gout, high blood pressure, and hay fever.

With all these doctors ordering all these drugs and tests, the risk for confusion seems overwhelming. So far, such problems have been relatively rare, in part because she is such an active and intelligent participant in her own care. When a physician's words or prescriptions do not make sense to her, SC does not hesitate to speak up. Inevitably, though, chaos sometimes creeps in.

Her Boston physicians might repeat a test already done in Rhode Island, because it is easier to duplicate the test than track the results down. The findings on a CT scan *done* in Boston by one physician are not communicated to the other doctors in either state. A medication prescribed by one doctor has a potentially dangerous interaction with a drug prescribed by another. A simple question—"Why am I coughing?"—can go unanswered for months. Each specialist tells her that the cough is not due to a problem in his or her area; no one addresses her issue.

In many ways, her medical story captures what is so right about U.S. medicine today—and what is so wrong. Without all those doctors, tests, and prescriptions, her problems would surely be worse. She would probably not be alive at age eighty, let alone reading the *New York Times* and making local politicians squirm.

SC is benefiting tremendously from modern medicine, but that benefit comes with a struggle that is at times harrowing. She feels like her medical care is a train that could go off the tracks at any time if she relaxes her guard. She knows that her care is less efficient, less reliable, and more hazardous than it should be. But like most patients, SC does not know what she or anyone else can do to assure that nothing slips through the cracks.

Failing Grades

The chaos that threatens the care of this patient and so many others may not be apparent from the statistics that describe the U.S. health care system. But the cumulative impact of the problems experienced by individuals like her is a health care system that is the most expensive in the world, yet so far from what one would expect in safety and reliability.

Concern that the U.S. health care system has fundamental problems has been building for decades, but the need for fundamental change is a relatively recent insight. The Institute of Medicine sounded the alarm in 2000 with the release of *To Err Is Human* [1]. This first report in a highly influential series focused on problems in patient safety, and described an epidemic of medical errors causing an estimated forty-four thousand to ninety-eight thousand deaths in the United States per year. The enduring image from that report was of a 747 airplane full of patients dying every day because of preventable medical injuries. The second report, released the next year, was titled *Crossing the Quality Chasm* [2]. This report described problems not just in patient safety but also in efficiency, timeliness, and the reliability with which care that is known to be helpful to patients is actually delivered.

In the years since, the gap between the health care we expect and what we actually receive has been characterized in painful detail. The research study that best captured the magnitude of the problem was published in the *New England Journal of Medicine* in 2003 by a research team led by Elizabeth McGlynn, from the California think tank known as RAND [3]. This study has been so influential that it is routinely quoted by candidates for political office in their critiques of the U.S. health care system.

McGlynn's team interviewed 13,275 randomly selected adults in twelve U.S. metropolitan areas. For about half of these people, the researchers obtained their actual medical records. Using these data, they were able to calculate how often people with thirty different medical conditions received tests and treatments that were likely to be beneficial. The study's "bottom line" became famous: the patients received only 54.9 percent of the interventions recommended for their conditions (e.g., eye exams for patients with diabetes).

Even when "the right thing" *usually* occurred, the gap between 100 percent reliability and the actual rate was surprising. Just 66 percent of recommended immunizations and 69 percent of recommended drugs were given, and patients with breast cancer received only 76 percent of recommended care interventions. For many everyday medical issues, the chances that the right thing happened seemed a coin flip—or worse. The weakest area was counseling or educating patients, which medical records suggested occurred only 18 percent of the times when it would be expected. Only 10.5 percent of the interventions for patients for alcohol dependence were documented as delivered.

One would expect that many medical interventions should be about as routine as airplane pilots putting down landing gear as they approach the ground, but here are the frequencies with which they actually occurred in the McGlynn study:

• Follow-up of the finding of a breast mass with further testing or a doctor visit within three months: 89 percent

• Performance of mammography annually in women with a history of breast cancer: 85 percent

• Use of aspirin within one week for patients with newly diagnosed coronary artery disease: 51 percent

• Use of insulin therapy in diabetic patients who have not achieved good control of their blood sugar levels with oral medications: 39 percent

At first, many people thought that the 55 percent finding had to be wrong, or that it must reflect poor care for socioeconomically disadvantaged Americans. But the results have been meticulously reviewed, and if anything, they understate the real gaps in quality. The good news–bad news story turns out to be that poor or nonwhite people have not cornered the market on mediocre health care. Whites were actually slightly *less* likely to receive recommended interventions than blacks or Hispanics. People with college or graduate school degrees received 56 percent of the interventions—about the same as the 55 percent rate for those who did not complete high school. Annual income, type of health insurance, age, and gender didn't matter much either.

According to this study, a fifty-year-old white female college graduate with private health insurance and a household income above $50,000 would receive 57 percent of the recommended care [4]. On the other hand, a fifty-year-old uninsured black man with less than a high school education and an income under $15,000 would receive 51 percent of the recommended care. The difference in quality experienced by these two types of patients was trivial compared to the gap between ideal care and reality. These two people might never cross paths in U.S. society, but they were likely to receive the same mediocre health care.

A more global look at the "opportunities for improvement" for the U.S. health care system was provided in 2006 by the Commonwealth Fund Commission on a High Performance Health System [5] and updated in 2008 [6]. Instead of comparing U.S. performance for various medical interventions to a theoretical ideal rate of 100 percent, this commission used real-world benchmarks—the rates achieved by other countries, or the top 10 percent of U.S. states, hospitals, health plans, or other groups of health care providers. Thus, the U.S. health care system was evaluated using real-world goals that fell well short of perfection. Think of this approach as grading the U.S. health care system on a curve.

Using this approach, the performance of the U.S. health care system averaged only 66 percent of the benchmark rates in 2006, and it had not improved at all in the 2008 update. The United States in fact fell from fifteenth to last place out of nineteen countries on a measure of mortality amenable to medical care, because other countries had improved while the U.S. performance stayed about the same. Compared with other countries, U.S. patients were less likely to have their medications reviewed at discharge or to report good access to care when they needed it. U.S. patients were also more likely to report medical, medication, or lab test errors.

The "underuse" of beneficial care may be particularly galling to physicians, because it reveals a lack of reliability that belies their public image. But there are two other major types of errors that are of comparable social concern. "Overuse" occurs when an intervention's benefits do not justify its potential harm or costs—for example, the performance of a high-cost radiology test that is unlikely to change a patient's treatment, or a prescription of antibiotics for a patient who probably has a viral respiratory infection. Although physicians may not set out to give treatments of little value to their patients, after-the-fact reviews of cases suggest that as many as one-third of some medical interventions may be clinically inappropriate [7]. The third type of error is "misuse," which occurs when a preventable complication eliminates the benefit of an intervention. An example is an allergic reaction to penicillin in a patient with a known allergy to this class of antibiotic.

Concern about overuse is driven by rising health care costs, while worries about misuse rise with each press report of patients who receive the wrong drug, have surgery on the wrong site, or have treatment complications that might have been foreseen and prevented. For patients, the impression that U.S. health care is dangerous is reinforced by their actual experiences. In one survey, more than a third of physicians and laypersons reported that there had been errors in their own care or a family member's care [8].

Critics of U.S. health care tend to focus on one issue at a time—for instance, our high costs, lack of safety, or lack of reliability. Perhaps because these challenges seem so formidable, health care leaders tend to specialize in one or at most two of these areas, as if they were separate battles to be fought. Responsibility for patient safety, cost reduction, and clinical quality improvement in hospitals may be assigned to three different people.

The wisdom and effectiveness of this division of labor are uncertain. A credible case can be made that these problems share the same root problem: medicine has become too complex for the way we deliver health care.

The Overwhelmed Physician

Although medicine has advanced rapidly in recent decades, the daily lives of many physicians have changed surprisingly little. They rise early, often before the sun is up, and go first to the hospital, where they see their patients who are hospitalized. They write (by hand usually) orders for the tests to be performed and treatments to be delivered that day. By 8:00 or 9:00 a.m. they are at their offices, where they are the only physician or perhaps one of two to three doctors. They work hard throughout the day, seeing patients every fifteen minutes or so. They write prescriptions for medications on paper prescription pads. In between patients, they make or take calls from patients, pharmacies, and colleagues. Then at night they carry home a stack of paperwork to be completed by the next day, when the cycle begins anew.

The pace of the physician's day has always been relentless, frequently hectic, but doctors have been sustained through the ages by something beyond monetary reward. They are respected throughout their communities—even romanticized for their selfless dedication to their patients. The cultural role of physicians is that of the heroic healer, sacrificing their own lives after a fashion to help patients extend theirs. Rising from bed in the middle of the night is just one more way in which physicians convey their commitment to patients. Indeed, appearing gaunt and exhausted has never been a professional liability for physicians.

Dedication is an expectation with which most physicians remain comfortable; more problematic is the related assumption that they are also all knowing. The rigors of medical training are hardly exaggerated in films and books. Of the 148 hours in a week, medical students and young physician trainees might spend 40 of them asleep, and devote virtually all the rest of those hours to learning their craft. At the end of their training, they assume a status in which their orders and advice are rarely questioned.

The special role of physicians as all-knowing healers is sustained partly because many patients harbor hopes that their doctors have near-magical powers. For example, one study found that about one-third of patients want to be on an equal footing with their physicians— such as calling each other by their first names. But a comparable percentage *want* to call their physicians by their title and last name (e.g., Dr. Smith), just as they also want their physicians to wear white coats [9]. As one psychiatrist-colleague puts it, "When people are sick, they don't want to put their fate in the hands of someone who could be sitting on the bar stool next to them later that evening. They don't want a friend—they want a healer who will cure them. They want someone with superhuman powers, so they don't really want to relate to physicians as equals."

This special status for physicians is established in subtle ways. Office staffs in many physician practices do not address physicians by their first names in front of patients. First-year medical students at over a hundred U.S. medical schools have "White Coat Ceremonies," in which they don the traditional physician garb with the solemnity of judges putting on robes. Some physicians (including one of the authors) were trained never to open a book to look up information in front of a patient, but to instead leave the room to find the needed facts. The unspoken message to patients is, "I have everything up here in my head."

This myth has proven unsustainable, however, and if there ever was a time when physicians really could keep everything they needed to know inside their heads, that era ended long ago. Since World War II, U.S. federal and corporate funding for research has grown rapidly, leading to not just new drugs and technologies but also an explosion in medical knowledge. According to the U.S. National Library of Medicine, there were 670,943 new articles that were indexed in 2007 in its database called MEDLINE—about twice as many as the 336,000 new articles published back in the Dark Ages of 1996 [10]. (The number of articles *retracted* because of errors or scientific fraud increased from 16 to 124 over that same period.)

A generation ago, physicians mastered their fields by reading textbooks like *Harrison's Principles of Internal Medicine* cover to cover. As the expansion of scientific knowledge accelerated, physicians came to rely on weekly periodicals such as the *New England Journal of Medicine* and regular hospital teaching conferences called Grand Rounds. Today's physicians feel so hopeless about their ability to keep up with the progress of medicine that many have given up on lifelong learning activities. Around the country, attendance at hospital teaching conferences is in decline, and subscriptions to medical journals have fallen off.

Many older physicians still struggle to stay current with medical science by continuing these time-honored educational activities, but younger physicians know that the game has changed. Instead, they seek to master tools that enable them to acquire knowledge "just-in-time" via the Internet. Many physicians use Google and Wikipedia to help them find the most current information, often right in front of their patients.

Even with all these resources, physicians are increasingly aware that as individuals, they cannot know everything they need to deliver state-of-the-science care, particularly for more complex patients with diseases of multiple systems. One direct result of the growth of medical knowledge is thus the emerging importance of specialty care (e.g., cardiology and oncology), and the division of specialists into finer and finer subcategories. At many academic medical centers, specialists focus on one problem and one problem only. For example, cardiologists are divided into experts on arrhythmia, heart failure, coronary disease, or prevention. Oncologists at major medical centers concentrate on just one disease—lymphoma experts do not see myeloma patients, and myeloma experts do not see Hodgkin's disease patients, and so on.

All this superspecialization is wonderful when the right patient gets to the right doctor. If you have multiple myeloma, you probably *do* want to have a doctor whose professional life is completely focused on that disease. Having such a physician will increase the chances that you get the most current therapy, and that he or she will recognize unusual complications or developments right away. For occasional patients, having that superspecialist might be the difference between survival and premature death.

On the other hand, the superspecialization of medicine can cause new challenges for patients and clinicians. One is that sick patients often have to see multiple physicians, particularly if they have multiple diseases. Consider the twelve physicians seen by SC in 2007 alone at a Boston teaching hospital fifty miles away from her home. In her case, the physicians all used the same electronic medical record (EMR), but 20 percent of U.S. physicians were using electronic records at that time [11], and few of these electronic records are able to communicate with each other. If her physicians had not all been at one institution, what are the chances that each of them would have known what the others were doing and thinking?

Another type of problem that is especially frustrating to patients arises when they have diseases or symptoms that do not fit cleanly into the domains of superspecialized physicians. These specialists may be extremely competent in their narrow area, but extremely uncomfortable outside of it. As a result, they approach patients considering the well-contained issue of "Is this what I do?" rather than the more ambitious question of "What is wrong?"

A joke in medicine is that young physicians who want to be on the cutting edge of medicine today should try to learn more and more about less and less, until they know everything about nothing. Conversely, doctors who want to be generalists, such as internists and other primary care physicians, are doomed to knowing less and less about more and more, until they know nothing about everything.

This joke reflects a major worrisome trend in modern medicine: primary care is losing its appeal to physicians, even as the subspecialization of medicine makes the coordinating role of a primary care doctor all the more essential. Complicated patients need *someone* who is focused on them as people as opposed to the diseases that they have. Nevertheless, among third-year internal medicine residents in 2003, only 27 percent planned to practice general medicine—a rate just half that of 1998 [12]. Young physicians are instead choosing careers with narrower scopes of knowledge and higher compensation.

The gap in pay between primary care physicians and specialists might matter more to young physicians in the United States than in other countries because U.S. doctors tend to graduate from medical school with so much debt. In many other countries, physicians have lower incomes, but medical school is completely or heavily subsidized by the government. In the United States, the median debt for physicians on graduation from medical school ranges from $115,000 at public institutions to $150,000 at private institutions [13]. Typical loan repayment rates are about $1,500 per month—an obligation that encourages young physicians to think long and hard about specialties that might pay two- to threefold more, even if they are attracted to primary care.

But money is not the only reason that primary care is losing its attraction. Data on the career choices of medical students who graduated from 1996 to 2002 suggest that a "controllable" lifestyle is more important than income or any other factor [14]. Table 1.1 shows how the researchers categorized each of sixteen specialty options on how controllable or "uncontrollable" a lifestyle they permitted, along with the average income, hours of work per week, and years of graduate medical education required. Primary care specialties, such as family practice, internal medicine, and pediatrics, were considered to have uncontrollable lifestyles. So were surgical specialties, but note that the average income of the uncontrollable surgical specialties was considerably higher than the primary care options. The detailed statistical analyses indicated that several factors influenced medical student career choices, including income, work hours, and years of training. None of these factors, however, were as critical as the appeal of a controllable lifestyle.

Table 1.1
Characteristics of the selected specialties

Specialty	Lifestyle	Average income, $ in thousands	Average work hours per week	Years of graduate medical education required
Anesthesiology	Controllable	225	61.0	
Dermatology	Controllable	221	45.5	4
Emergency medicine	Controllable	183	46.0	4
Family practice	Uncontrollable	132	52.5	3
Internal medicine	Uncontrollable	158	57.0	3
Neurology	Controllable	172	55.5	4
Obstetrics and gynecology	Uncontrollable	224	61.0	4
Ophthalmology	Controllable	225	47.0	4
Orthopedic surgery	Uncontrollable	323	58.0	5
Otolaryngology	Controllable	242	53.5	5
Pathology	Controllable	202	45.5	4
Pediatrics	Uncontrollable	138	54.0	3
Psychiatry	Controllable	134	48.0	4
Radiology (diagnostic)	Controllable	263	58.0	4
Surgery (general)	Uncontrollable	238	60.0	5
Urology	Uncontrollable	245	60.5	5
Average for the above specialties	Not applicable	208	53.9	4

What does a controllable lifestyle mean? In this study, having control over one's work hours was critical to the definition, and other data confirm that younger physicians place a high priority on time for life outside work. These priorities are somewhat in conflict with the concept of the selfless physician willing to be there for his or her patient at any time or place. Still, these priorities are consistent with a modern society in which many physicians' households have two working adults, and about half of graduating physicians are women, many of whom expect to start families. The incomes in these households are substantial—but life itself does not feel, well, controllable.

Of course, these issues are not restricted to medicine. Families with two highly educated spouses with demanding careers are part of a national trend that has seen the proportion of married employees in dual-earner couples rise from 66 percent in 1977 to 78 percent in 2002 [15]. Noting an increasing tendency toward educational parity between spouses, one report on these workforce trends concluded that "families have now reached their limits. They have no more hours available to add to the labor force or to improve family income. . . . Higher educated employees under onerous time demands face the need to gain greater flexibility and control over how, when, and how long they work. Young professionals, particularly women, need to be able to reduce their working hours, to allow them to remain in the careers their education has prepared them to pursue" [16].

Now here is the truly troubling news. If the problems with primary care were just the pay and the demanding hours, they might be addressed by expensive yet simple measures like paying primary care doctors more and reducing the number of patients that they see. The conviction is growing, though, that the problem with primary care may be the job itself.

Primary care physicians are no longer the all-knowing healers of a generation ago. Instead, they spend much of their day managing an overwhelming flow of information—lab tests; requests for referrals, prescriptions, and the completion of forms; calls from patients and family members. Various studies have found that a typical primary care physician spends an average of seventy-four minutes per day reviewing test results [17], and has to review an estimated eight hundred chemistry and hematology reports, forty radiology reports, and twelve pathology reports per week [18]. The risk of an error is ever present; in one study, 83 percent of physicians reported that there had been at least one test result they wish they had known about sooner during the previous two months [17].

Besides having too much patient data to track, there is, quite simply, too much to know—even for the bread-and-butter issues that dominate the life of primary care doctors. Take one of the most mundane problems in medicine: the simple urinary tract infection. A generation ago, there were perhaps two to three options for treating these infections; today there are dozens. Physicians hesitate when prescribing drugs they have been using for years, wondering if they are giving their patient the best treatment possible, in the right dose, for the right number of days.

Similarly, when physicians in their fifties and sixties went to medical school, there was one test for diagnosing pulmonary embolism; there are now at least five tests that are commonly used, in a wide array of combinations. Hepatitis B was an easy problem for the physician in those days—there was no treatment. But at present about seven different drugs are effective, and only specialists in this condition are comfortable prescribing them. For any given issue or any given drug, physicians have the ability to learn the state of the art—in theory. In reality, there are too many issues and too many drugs, and not enough time to learn about them. Being human, many physicians do not know where to begin.

A painful irony, therefore, is that the increase in our collective knowledge causes individual physicians to feel less knowledgeable. Medicine's ability to help patients is expanding, but physicians' comfort zones are shrinking—especially in primary care. In a large survey in the 1990s, 24 percent of primary care physicians reported that the "scope of care" they were expected to provide was greater than it should be [19]. There is no particular reason to suspect that this percentage has decreased.

Meanwhile, the number of tests performed, drugs being used, and specialists being consulted all continue to rise, and the primary care physician is expected to know and coordinate everything. In the paper-based world of most physician offices, this effort is not going well. In a 2003 study of thirty-two primary care clinics in Colorado, primary care physicians reported that they were missing important clinical information in 14 percent of the visits [20]. The missing data included laboratory results (6 percent of all visits); letters or dictations (5 percent), radiology results (4 percent), history and physical examinations (4 percent), and medication information (3 percent). The physicians believed the missing data were at least somewhat likely to adversely affect their patients in about 44 percent of the cases, and reported spending significant time unsuccessfully trying to track down the data (five to ten minutes, 26 percent; more than ten minutes, 10 percent).

Physicians hate to make mistakes, but even with superhuman efforts, they cannot always avoid them. A typical primary care doctor follows a panel of twenty-five hundred patients. Some experts calculate that a typical group of patients of that size requires 7.4 hours of physician time per day for basic preventive services, and another 10.6 hours per day for the care of common chronic disease [21, 22]. If these estimates are correct, physicians are either not getting enough sleep or not doing everything that their own guidelines suggest they should do. Both are probably true.

The missed opportunities to give patients care that would be beneficial to them (the 55 percent phenomenon) may be a relatively benign
form of failure. More horrifying are the times when doctors prescribe
drugs that potentially endanger patients because patients are allergic
to the medications or because the drugs may interact with other medications being used by the patient. How often does this occur? One
study found that for every one hundred Medicare enrollees per year,
there is a rate of five "adverse events" from medications, of which more
than one-fourth were preventable [23].

Doctors still work long days, but primary care physicians in particular say that they leave work at the end of those days feeling that their
work is not complete. They worry that they have made mistakes
because there were things they should have known yet did not, or
things that they just did not get to.

A Loss of Trust

Doctors are not the only people who are worried. The general public
is bombarded by information about hazards to health from every angle,
including the news media, direct-to-consumer advertising, and medical
dramas on television. This information is irresistibly interesting, almost
hypnotic. For example, CNN has actively solicited cancer survivor
stories to share with others in a feature called *Saving Your Life* [24].

Even when the information in the media is accurate, it is often difficult for consumers to place in perspective. The fact is that the organizations (including health care providers) that offer this information
have business interests that are served by arousing a certain amount of
alarm. For better *and* worse, U.S. consumers are being turned into
patients. They are forced into awareness of the diseases and aging
processes that might compromise their health, and wonder if they are
getting everything they could and should.

One thing is clear: Americans *are* getting a lot of health care, and the
amount is increasing. Prescription drug use rose from about 4 drugs
per person in 1994 to 5.2 drugs in 2001–2002 [25], and the number of
X-rays and other tests performed continues to rise at a similar pace.
Some of these increases represent real progress that helps people live
longer and better lives, but many prescriptions are written and tests
ordered to provide peace of mind to patients who are worried.

When people worry, they question relationships that were trusting
in the past, and the doctor-patient relationship is no exception. An

analysis of survey data collected from 1976 to 1998 showed that physicians are still held in relatively high regard by the general public, but there was an erosion of trust and respect for doctors during this period [26]. Since a major component of career satisfaction for physicians is their stature in the community, the importance of this erosion is clear. Physicians mourn the loss of trust, and a vicious cycle is set in motion, since physicians who are walking (or running) around in a foul mood do not inspire confidence in patients that the health care system is going to meet their needs.

The facts sometimes tell a story quite different from general impressions. For example, physicians *and* patients believe that visits with doctors have gotten shorter and shorter. And it would make sense if this were actually true. The number of patient visits to physicians' offices has been steadily rising [27], and physicians have squeezed more and more visits in per day because of rising demand from patients and financial pressures. Paperwork and other tasks that must occur outside the visit (e.g., communicating with the many other doctors participating in a complex patient's care or entering data in computerized medical records) have only increased. So face-to-face time with patients must be decreasing, right?

Not so, at least according to data from two large surveys that studied office visits in large samples of U.S. physician practices. One survey found that the average duration of the visit increased by 1.1 minutes from 1989 to 1998, while the other reported a 2.0-minute increase. The increases in visit duration were found for primary care and specialist physicians, managed care and non-managed care patients, and new patients and return visits [27].

If doctors are spending more time with patients, why does it seem like less? There is just so much more to do than a generation ago. To take good care of patients today, physicians need to keep track of vaccinations to reduce their patients' risks of influenza and pneumonia, and tests to screen them for cancer and risk factors for cardiovascular disease. Conversations that often last several minutes are needed to explain options for screening patients for prostate cancer ("Is a prostate-specific antigen test really a good idea?"), colon cancer (colonoscopy versus home testing kits, versus other options), and atherosclerosis ("Should I have an exercise test, a CT scan, or a new special blood test?") Physicians are urged to screen patients for depression, alcohol abuse, and domestic violence. A good breast examination takes several minutes. Patients' expectations that their physicians will do all these things are high; after all, those patients have been learning what to expect from the media.

All available data indicate that despite the slightly longer visits, patients' expectations are often not met, and that the care they receive seems inefficient, poorly coordinated, and unsafe. The 2008 Commonwealth Fund Survey of Public Views of the U.S. Health Care System [28] found the following when it asked adults to describe their health care experiences during the previous two years:

- Physicians ordered a test that had already been done: 17 percent
- Patients had difficulty getting advice from physicians during regular office hours: 41 percent
- Physicians failed to provide important medical history or test results to other doctors or nurses: 21 percent

Other data show that 31 percent of sicker adults report that during the past two years, they had left a doctor's office without getting crucial questions answered, and 39 percent reported that they did not follow a doctor's advice [29]. In another study, just 51 percent of the people surveyed felt that their primary care physicians' knowledge of their entire medical history was excellent or very good, and just 36 percent thought their doctors had excellent or very good knowledge of what worried them most about their health [30]. Of senior citizens who reported in a national survey that they had skipped doses or stopped medications because of side effects or their belief that the medication was not working, 39 percent had not talked with a physician about it [31].

Like so many other components of modern medicine, the doctor-patient relationship is under duress.

The picture we have painted is one of a health care system that feels out of control to patients and the physicians caring for them. It is a system that is failing to meet the needs of patients with reliability, where no one—the doctors, the patients, and the parties paying for health care—is happy or believes the status quo is sustainable. Before contemplating solutions, we will next examine the forces that created the chaos that threatens health care.

2 Progress

Health care has its share of "bad guys" who warrant criticism—including businesses reaping exorbitant profits, criminals who commit fraud, and physicians who practice sloppy medicine, to name a few. And our challenges would be simpler if the driving force behind U.S. health care's problems was the greed or incompetence of these people. We could round the culprits up and put them out of business.

Unfortunately, we cannot lock up the dominant force behind rising health care costs, and even if we could, we would not want to. That force is progress itself—technological innovations like new drugs that make incurable diseases curable; new tests that hasten diagnosis and reduce uncertainty; and new surgical techniques that lead to shorter recovery periods.

When used correctly on the right patients, these innovations can mean a longer and better life, peace of mind, or at least the knowledge needed to make informed decisions. But these innovations also generate costs and confusion. Increasingly sophisticated care requires sophisticated specialists who immerse themselves in narrow areas of medicine. That trend inevitably means more physicians must be involved in the care of complex patients, with more opportunities for miscommunication and inefficiency.

In this chapter, we examine the role of several factors that are often blamed for the crisis in health care and explore how the ongoing explosion of medical knowledge leads to the chaos described in chapter 1. We believe that regardless of how health care is financed, the management of information and choices created by medical progress is a challenge that must be addressed. We also believe that this challenge is surmountable. Before we can imagine the "cure," however, we must understand the "disease process" at work.

Why Are Health Care Costs Rising?

Let's focus for now on rising costs as the destabilizing issue in health care, and temporarily put aside concerns about quality and safety. After all, if health care is unaffordable, patients cannot get access to care, and quality and safety concerns become academic.

Let's also temporarily put aside the issue of the high *baseline* level of U.S. health care spending compared to other countries. Many other books and articles look at issues such as what percentage of U.S. gross domestic product devoted to health care is sustainable, the percentage of health care spending attributable to the "overhead" of a fragmented multipayer health care system, and the higher prices of everything in U.S. health care from pharmaceuticals to personnel.

For the moment, though, we would like to concentrate on the factors driving the *increases* in health care costs, because it is those annual increases of 7 to 12 percent that disrupt the budgets of employers, individuals, and government. All of these budgets seem stretched to the limit right now, and the knowledge that they will be stretched even more next year by higher health care costs induces a sense of panic.

What can possibly cause increases that have averaged about 9 percent per year for such a large industry over the past quarter century [1]? The usual suspects are:

- Rising pharmaceutical and device prices
- Administrative costs of the health care system
- Medical malpractice
- Aging of the population
- Behavioral and lifestyle choices
- Hospital and physician costs
- Technological innovations
- More frequent use of older tests and therapies

All of these factors contribute to the high baseline cost of health care, but some of them are surprisingly unimportant as drivers of *growth* in overall health care spending.

A thorough and objective examination of the drivers of increases in health care costs was presented in a January 2008 Congressional Budget Office (CBO) paper titled *Technological Change and the Growth of Health Care Spending* [2]. The CBO paper confirms that the United States

Table 2.1
Average real growth of health care expenditures, 2005

Country	Average real annual growth (percent)		
	1975–1985	1985–1995	1995–2005
United States	4.9	4.2	3.7
Luxembourg	3.9	4.9	8.4
Norway	4.6	3.8	6.6
Switzerland	2.3	2.5	2.9
Austria	1.5	6.0	2.5
Iceland	5.4	1.7	4.3
Belgium	4.1	3.4	4.3
France	4.2	3.6	3.0
Canada	3.5	1.8	2.9
Germany	2.8	1.7	2.0
Australia	1.5	2.3	4.8*
Netherlands	1.4	3.1	4.1*
Denmark	2.2	0.9	3.3
Sweden	2.5	0	3.3
United Kingdom	2.4	3.6	4.9
Italy	N.A.	1.3**	2.9
Japan	4.5	2.6	2.9*

Source: CBO based on data from the Organisation for Economic Co-operation and Development ([2], 5). Spending amounts are adjusted for inflation using the gross domestic product implicit price deflator from the Bureau of Economic Analysis. N.A. = not available.
*Data are for 1995–2004
**Data are for 1988–1995

spends more on health care per person than do other industrialized countries, but notes that other countries have had about the same rate of increase. Table 2.1 shows the CBO's analysis of the average annual growth by country from 1975 to 1995. In summarizing the context for its analysis, the CBO paper says, "Although growth rates vary by country and by period, most industrialized countries—*even those with a financing system quite different from that in the United States*—have experienced a substantial long-term rise in real spending on health care. In fact, growth rates in per capita spending in some countries have exceeded those in the United States during some periods" ([2], 3–4; emphasis added).

An analysis of expenditure patterns for various categories of health care provides insight into why many of the usual suspects have less

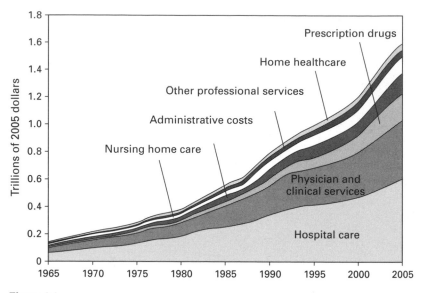

Figure 2.1
Real spending on health care in selected categories, 1965–2005. CBO analysis based on data on spending on health services and supplies, as defined in the national health expenditure accounts, maintained by the Centers for Medicare and Medicaid Services. Spending amounts are adjusted for inflation using the gross domestic product implicit price deflator from the Bureau of Economic Analysis. (*Source*: [2])

impact on cost increases than one would expect. Figure 2.1 from the CBO report shows that the dominant sectors and areas of growth in health care spending during the last century have been hospitals, physicians, and other clinical services. Expenditures on administrative costs and prescription drugs have increased, but these categories remain relatively minor. For example, the pharmaceutical industry's portion of health care spending is about 10 percent. Price increases and high profit margins in this sector alone cannot be major drivers of rising overall health care costs. Even if these companies were nationalized and their profits eliminated, overall health care spending would fall by just 1 to 2 percent.

Administrative expenses generated by commercial insurance plans are another tempting target. These costs rose at about 14 percent per year from 1997 to 2003—well above the overall rate of increase in health care spending [3]. Still, administrative overhead is only 7 percent of the total U.S. health care spending, so even this rate of increase cannot explain a major portion of the overall growth of expenditures.

The medical malpractice system is often blamed for rising health care costs, particularly by physicians. It raises expenses in two ways: the premiums that physicians must pay for malpractice insurance, and the tests and treatments that physicians order not because they believe the patient needs them but rather to provide them with protection against a malpractice suit. These extra tests and treatments are frequently described as "defensive medicine." Ironically, they actually offer little protection against malpractice suits. Most successful suits are based on physician failures to communicate with colleagues or the patient, or to follow through with standard care ("dropped balls" such as the failure to react to an abnormal mammogram).

Concerns about malpractice do contribute to test utilization, so that the expenses attributable to medical malpractice are increasing at about 12 percent per year. Yet the *total* cost of medical liability and defensive medicine are estimated to account for just 10 percent of the overall health care spending [4]. Thus, even with a 12 percent rate of rise, the malpractice system is a trivial force in the growth in health care costs.

The aging of the baby boomers is a powerful trend that will have major impacts on health care in the decades ahead, but the available data indicate that demographic trends explain only a small portion of the annual increases in spending [1, 2]. The CBO estimates that changes in the age distribution from 1965 to 2005 account for just 3 percent of the cumulative increases in health care spending that occurred during that period [2]. The explanation for this paradox is as follows: the aging of the population is a slow process akin to global warming. As in the case with climate change, the average age of the population is only slightly higher in any given year than it was the year before. Between 2005 and 2015, the average age of the U.S. population is projected to increase from 36.5 to 37.9—an average per year increase of only 0.37 percent [5].

Several other factors blunt the cost impact of the growing proportion of the population that is elderly [1]. Per capita spending for the elderly is increasing more slowly than per capita spending for the nonelderly. The elderly are living longer, but the average number of years of disability is actually decreasing, which decreases the cost impact of greater life expectancy. Finally, considerable spending occurs at the end of life, but these costs are not rising faster than health expenditures as a whole.

Just as some climate change experts worry that global warming could accelerate in the years ahead, we should note that as the baby boomers age, there could be an acceleration of health care spending for the elderly that goes beyond the increase in the number of senior citizens. This generation has higher expectations than its predecessors for physical function, and can be expected to try to slow deterioration through procedures like knee, back, and shoulder surgery. They are overweight and getting heavier, which is leading to increasing rates of diabetes, hypertension, heart attacks, and heart failure. And they do not seem particularly inclined to be philosophical about the inevitable approach of the end of life—that is, they may tend to want to try every possible treatment, even when the outlook seems hopeless.

The increased *utilization* of health care by the baby boomers and everyone else is driving increased spending in the two largest sectors: hospitals and physicians. Nevertheless, an increase in *prices* due to higher wages is not a major force behind rising health care costs, with one major exception. The general shortage of nurses combined with the growing technical sophistication of the nursing required by high-tech medicine have led to substantial wage increases for nurses, whose salaries account for about 30 percent of most hospitals' budgets. Other health care personnel, however, are generally receiving salary increases in line with consumer price inflation.

The nonpersonnel costs within hospitals and physicians' offices are rising due to growing investments in information systems, new technologies, and the infrastructure needed to support them. For example, operating rooms today need to be larger to accommodate robotics and other equipment required for minimally invasive surgery. Ceilings and walls in hospitals are torn out and even enlarged to accommodate the wiring of information systems. New facilities are being built so that patients with cancer and other previously untreatable conditions can receive advanced new medications that have to be given by intravenous lines.

This brings us back to the factor that is the major driver of cost increases across so many of sectors in figure 2.1: progress itself. After accounting for a range of issues affecting the demand for health care including increases attributable to the expansion of insurance coverage and personal income growth, economists believe that one-half to two-thirds of long-term spending growth reflects the "march of science" [2, 3]. The CBO report of January 2008 summarized three examinations of the drivers of growth in health care spending and found consistent conclusions to that effect (table 2.2). Progress in manufacturing industries usually drives down costs; why does it

Table 2.2

Estimated contributions of selected factors to long-term growth in real health care spending per capita, 1940 to 1990

	Smith, Heffler, and Freeland (2000)	Cutler (1995)	Newhouse (1992)
Aging of the population	2%	2%	2%*
Changes in third-party payment	10%	13%	10%
Personal income growth	11–18%	5%	<23%
Prices in the healthcare sector	11–22%	19%	Not estimated
Administrative costs	3–10%	13%	Not estimated
Defensive medicine and supplier-induced demand	0%	Not estimated	0%
Technology-related changes in medical practice	**38–62%**	**49%**	**≻65%**

Notes: Amounts in table represent the estimated percentage share of long-term growth that each factor accounts for.
*Data for 1950 to 1987
**Data for 1950 to 1980
Source: Congressional Budget Office [2] based on Smith SD, Keffler SK, Freeland MS, The impact of technological change on health care cost increases: An evaluation of the literature (working paper, 2000); Cutler DM, Technology, health costs, and the NIH (paper prepared for the National Institutes of Health Economics Roundtable on Biomedical Research, September 1995); Newhouse JR, Medical care costs: How much welfare loss? *Journal of Economic Perspectives* 1992;6:3–22.

increase expenditures in health care? A critical distinction is that in health care, the "product" is constant changing. Thomas Bodenheimer cites the example of treatment of acute myocardial infarction, which as recently as 1980 was treated with a week of bed rest in the coronary care unit and a limited array of medications [6]. Today, the total hospital length of stay for patients with acute myocardial infarction is often just a few days, but they may undergo cardiac catheterization, coronary angioplasty with stents costing $2,000 per vessel, treatment with bioengineered drugs to dissolve blood clots, and coronary artery bypass graft surgery. They are sent home on a variety of medications that help them live longer by lowering adrenaline levels (beta-blockers), reducing cholesterol (statins), and preventing blood clots (aspirin and many times clopidogrel). The result has been a much greater chance of surviving for patients with heart attacks, but also much higher costs.

Hopes that progress may reduce costs have thus far been unfilled, and are likely to remain that way. Most medical advances lead to better patient outcomes, but at a higher cost per patient. Even when advances lower the cost of treating individual patients, spending can be expected to increase. As in other sectors of the economy, when the unit cost of a good decreases, the number of people who purchase that product increases, so that net spending tends to go up. A frequently cited example of a technology that lowered costs but increased spending is laparoscopic cholecystectomy, which costs about 25 percent less than the older procedure for removing gall bladders and requires a much shorter recovery time. The newer, cheaper, and less painful procedure has been applied to a much larger patient population, so that overall spending on cholecystectomy has increased [7].

Other examples abound in which newer, less expensive, and less painful procedures have been introduced—and are then used to treat an expanded patient population so that the net spending increases. These instances include coronary angioplasty, knee arthroscopy, and laparoscopic gastric bypass surgery. As the knowledge needed to perform these procedures and tests becomes well established, they diffuse out from the teaching hospitals to lower-cost settings—community hospitals, ambulatory surgery centers, and physicians' offices—and beyond. With each step, the costs of providing the innovation decreases, but the overall spending on them increases.

Progress? What Progress?

Employers often complain that their health care costs go up every year and they do not get anything in return for the higher payments. Their distress is understandable, but their observation is wrong. Medical research is constantly producing new insights, new tests, and new treatments. Each year, the health care purchased with those insurance premiums is better than in the past. The difference may not be obvious from year to year, yet the progress is hard to miss with a longer perspective.

When we began our medical training in the 1960s and 1970s, for example, physicians could only guess at what disease processes might be causing neurological abnormalities such as a seizure or new weakness. But since the 1970s, we have witnessed the introduction of brain CT scanners that allowed the detection of tumors, strokes, and other diseases. In the decades that followed, MRI and PET scanners have come along, providing even more refined looks inside the body, while CT scanners have become so ubiquitous that many physician groups have them in their offices. In vitro fertilization was introduced in 1978, and today, one out of every fifty births in Sweden and one in eighty to a hundred births in the United States result from in vitro fertilization [8]. Bypass surgery for coronary artery disease became common, but then many patients who might have undergone bypass surgery instead had a lower cost and less uncomfortable procedure—balloon angioplasty. More recently, "plain old balloon angioplasty" (known as POBA among cardiologists) has given way to the use of metal coronary stents to hold open the arteries, and even *more* recently, "bare" metal stents have been replaced for many patients by stents coated with a variety of medications. The list of new drugs that have quickly become fixtures in U.S. medicine cabinets include statins for cholesterol reduction, ibuprofen and other anti-inflammatory agents, oral medications for the treatment of diabetes, and pills for erectile dysfunction, to name just a few.

Even with a shorter time frame, the impact of medical progress is startling. Until the introduction of highly active antiretroviral therapy in the mid-1990s, AIDS was virtually always a fatal disease with a life expectancy measured in months. The cultural impact of AIDS was partially captured by a pair of essays written a decade apart by Susan Sontag. In 1978, while she was being treated for breast cancer, she published *Illness as Metaphor*, in which she compared the experience of patients with cancer to those who suffered from tuberculosis, an incurable scourge that was often romanticized in nineteenth-century literature. A decade later, in 1988, Sontag wrote *AIDS and Its Metaphors*, in which she extended her comparisons to cancer to the dread surrounding AIDS. A decade after *that*, progress had made Sontag's insights on AIDS seem dated.

People with HIV infections who have access to the right medications have a near-normal life expectancy at present. This achievement did not come in one dramatic step but rather in a series of breakthroughs, each building on prior advances. HIV experts look back on the last two decades and see six different treatment eras [9]:

1. *1989* Drug treatment to reduce *pneumocystis jiroveci* pneumonia begins. Estimated per person survival benefit = 3.1 months.

2. *1993* Drug treatment to reduce infections with *Mycobacterium avium* complex disease. Estimated overall survival benefit of available treatments = 24.4 months.

3. *1996–1997 (ART 1)*   Introduction of potent combination antiretroviral therapy (ART) with the widespread use of drugs called protease inhibitors. Estimated overall survival benefit = 93.7 months.

4. *1998–1999 (ART 2)*   Sequential use of regimens called nonnucleoside reverse transcriptase inhibitors followed by protease inhibitors. Estimated overall survival benefit = 132.6 months.

5. *2000–2002 (ART 3)*   Three different effective regimens became available, with increased options for salvaging patients who were doing poorly. Estimated overall survival benefit = 138.8 months.

6. *2003 (ART 4)*   Improved drug efficacy with decreased side effects and regimen complexity as well as introduction of enfuvirtide. Estimated overall survival benefit = 159.9 months.

HIV is just one of the fields in which the pace of progress is accelerating. Insulin therapy for diabetes was introduced in 1921, and the next major breakthrough came in 1946, with the U.S. Food and Drug Administration (FDA) approval of the first oral medication (sulfonylureas) to lower blood sugar. A second oral medication (Metformin) was not approved by the FDA until 1995. But since then, the FDA has approved eight new antidiabetes medications as well as an insulin preparation that can be inhaled instead of injected via a needle [10].

The impact of progress is most readily evident in epidemiological data on heart disease, because heart disease is so common, and the impact of interventions can be measured in reductions in death rates (as opposed to harder-to-measure outcomes such as disability and the quality of life). Death rates from heart failure and heart attacks are going down in response to an array of drugs and devices that were merely good ideas a decade ago. One recent study analyzed data on 44,372 patients from around the world who were hospitalized with heart attacks or severe attacks of angina between July 1999 and December 2006 [11]. This paper found that the use of key medications (beta-blockers, statins, and angiotensin-converting enzyme inhibitors) and coronary angioplasty rose during this period, while the rate of death from heart attacks fell 18 percent.

The list of potential examples is long, and gets longer with each week's editions of the leading medical journals. Fibroid tumors in the uterus that cause bleeding and pain can often be treated by blocking blood vessels with special "catheters" (thin tubes) instead of hysterectomy [12]. Bariatric (weight loss) and heart valve replacement surgeries are being performed without any incisions in the skin. Genetic markers are being used to identify which therapies are most likely to benefit patients with lung and breast cancer. And the pace of progress is picking up.

How Progress Happens: A Case Study

What are the ingredients that produce progress in medicine? Bright people working hard with plentiful resources are a good start, but luck definitely plays a role. One of our favorite examples of a major medical advance shows that luck is important, though not random, and that the way in which health care is organized can increase the likelihood of progress.

This story begins in January 2002, when a woman named Kate Robbins developed a headache. A nurse in her midforties, she initially thought her headache was nothing more than postholiday stress. (Note: Robbins was the subject of a story on her remarkable case in the *Boston Globe* on November 24, 2003. Other patients mentioned in this book are all real, but are not identified by name.)

But this headache did not go away, so Robbins sought medical help. After a series of tests, she was found to have a tumor in her brain that had spread from a three-inch cancer in the upper part of her right lung. The best estimate of her life expectancy was eight to ten months.

Despite the poor prognosis, Robbins was not giving up. She had a family (her husband and two young children) that needed her. So she had surgery to remove the tumors in her brain and chest, and chemotherapy and radiation to try to kill the cancer cells remaining in her body. Nevertheless, her cancer spread to her liver and pancreas. Complications kept her in the hospital virtually the entire summer of 2002. As she told the *Boston Globe*, she started a journal of advice for her children on topics like dating and family—advice that she did not expect to be alive to give in person.

She was down to "last gasp" treatments that had not been shown to be effective in most patients. But Robbins was not your typical person with lung cancer. She was a relatively young woman who had never smoked cigarettes. And while it seems strange to describe someone with advanced lung cancer as lucky, that is exactly what she turned out to be. Robbins received a new treatment for lung cancer, and she had an extraordinary response: her cancer seemed to melt away.

The drug that she received is called gefitinib (made by Astra Zeneca under the name Iressa). It is among the first "smart drugs" that have been developed to treat cancer—ideally with more effectiveness and lower rates of complications. Traditional chemotherapy and radiation are more like weapons of mass destruction that damage all cells, regardless of whether they are normal or diseased. But Iressa was designed to attach itself to a target on the surface of lung cancer cells called epidermal growth factor receptor (EGFR), and then block the signals that tell tumors to grow and spread. In theory, Iressa should stop the growth of tumors without causing major side effects.

It was a wonderful idea. But like many great ideas, it did not actually work—at least not in most patients. In early clinical research trials, Iressa led to improvements in only 10 to 19 percent of the patients. Some of these patients, like Robbins, had *amazing* responses, but the overall assessment of Iressa was one of disappointment, since most patients did not benefit at all. Give the drug to a hundred patients with lung cancer, and they would not have a statistically better survival than a hundred patients who did not receive the drug. Therefore, the FDA approved Iressa for use only for lung cancer patients who had failed two attempts at treatment with other drugs or radiation—the traditional weapons of mass destruction.

Robbins was in that sad category when she received Iressa from a physician named Tom Lynch, MD, an oncologist at Massachusetts General Hospital (MGH) who specializes in lung cancer. A warm and friendly man who has witnessed more than his share of cancer tragedies, Lynch was ecstatic when Robbins turned out to be one of the winners in the Iressa lottery. Her tumors disappeared, and the *Boston Globe* ran a front-page story on Robbins and her seemingly miraculous cure.

That *Boston Globe* story caught the eye of *another* MGH physician, one who frequently crossed paths with Lynch but had never discussed Robbins or any other patient with him. That colleague was Daniel A. Haber, a physician who also has a PhD, and spends most of his day doing laboratory research on breast cancer, kidney cancer, and a variety of other malignancies—but *not* on lung cancer.

From that research, Haber knew that some cancers had genetic mutations that made the tumors especially vulnerable to new smart cancer drugs. He also knew how Iressa was designed to work. As he read the *Globe* article, he had a fleeting thought: he wondered if Robbins had some mutation in her cancer's version of EGFR that explained why her tumor seemed to dissolve when she received Iressa, when others did not benefit at all. But Haber is someone who comes up with such ideas all the time, and if he tried to explore every idea that occurred to him, he would have trouble getting anything done. So he turned the page of the newspaper and went on with his day.

That might have been the end of story. Soon after, though, Haber happened to have a few minutes to kill with Lynch. He knew Lynch from a weekly administration meeting of the MGH Hematology Oncology/Cancer Center, but they had never worked together in either patient care or research. Sipping coffee outside the conference room where that group met, he mentioned his idea to Lynch about an EGFR mutation as a possible explanation for why some patients responded so dramatically to Iressa. They decided to test the theory together.

Lynch rounded up tumor samples from nine patients who, like Robbins, were Iressa responders. Figure 2.2 shows a CT scan of the chest of one of those patients. On the left, nearly half of the chest is filled with the tumor. After treatment, most of the tumor has disappeared. The genetic findings from these nine tumors were compared with those from seven patients who did not respond to Iressa.

The laboratory research showed mutations of EGFR in eight of the nine responders, and none of the nonresponders. These mutations made EGFR about tenfold more sensitive to inhibition by Iressa—explaining why some patients like Robbins benefited so much from the drug, while most did not. They described their findings in a paper in

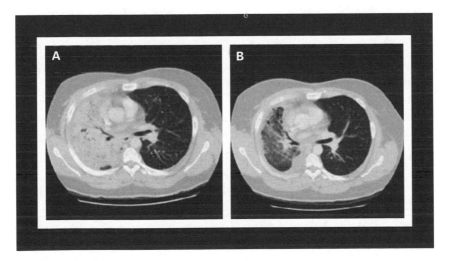

Figure 2.2
Example of the response to gefitinib in a patient with refractory non-small-cell lung cancer. (*Source*: [13])

the *New England Journal of Medicine* that has become one of the most widely cited research studies of the new century [13]. Subsequent research has shown that such tumor markers can identify patients who have about an 80 percent chance of responding to Iressa and drugs like it.

So many coincidences had to take place for this advance to occur when and how it did. Robbins had to seek care from Lynch, at a teaching hospital nearly an hour from home (on a good day given Boston traffic patterns), where just finding a parking space can be a challenge. Lynch had to know about Iressa, and feel comfortable trying this new medication on her. The *Boston Globe* had to find her story stirring. Haber had to notice the story and wonder whether a phenomenon observed in other cancers might be relevant. Haber and Lynch had to interact as part of their daily lives, and have a few moments for small talk. Lynch had to work in a setting where he could get his hands on tumors from nine Iressa responders.

Rather than focus on the serendipity behind this particular advance, however, one can examine the organizational factors that made it possible. After all, as the legendary French scientist Louis Pasteur said, chance favors the prepared mind. Lynch and Haber were prepared in part because they work in a community in which research is a passion, so they were ready to adapt knowledge from other diseases and explore whether this might somehow be relevant to patients like Robbins.

In a sense, the health care system worked perfectly in this case. Robbins was diagnosed, and her treatment was initiated. When her treatment was unsuccessful, she was referred to an academic medical center where physicians like Lynch see the most challenging cases. When something extraordinary happened in Robbins's case, the physicians around her were experienced enough to recognize it, sophisticated enough to think about it, and had the resources to explore it scientifically. An ideal health care system would be not only safe and efficient but also reliable in getting the Robbins of the world to doctors like Lynch and scientists like Haber.

Was this just an idea whose time had come? In a sense, yes. If Lynch and Haber had not had this flash of insight, someone else eventually would have. Indeed, as they were doing this work, researchers just across town at two other Harvard institutions, the Dana Farber Cancer Institute and the Brigham and Women's Hospital, came up with similar observations, which were published at nearly the same time in another journal. The pieces of the puzzle were ready to be assembled.

But those puzzles tend to get solved when the right people bump into each other at the right time in the right circumstances. If those interactions do not occur naturally and frequently, the era in which genetic markers help doctors choose better drugs for their patients with cancer and other diseases will be a little slower in arriving.

The Direct and Indirect Costs of Progress

That's the good news. The bad news, of course, is that creating progress is expensive, and so is paying for the tests and treatments that progress makes possible. Innovation can require high-stakes gambles of time and money. Estimates of the total cost of developing a novel drug are as high as $800 million, which is expended over a decade or more [14]. When the innovation is successful and leads to blockbuster drugs like statins, the reward for investors can be enormous. But more often than not, the gambles do not work out.

A spectacular example of a failed gamble was torcetrapib, a drug that seemed to offer the promise of preventing heart attacks by raising high-density lipoprotein cholesterol—also known as the "good cholesterol" because higher levels are associated with a reduced risk of heart disease. Pfizer spent fifteen years and nearly $1 billion to develop and test this drug in research studies around the world. The initial results were promising, and everyone expected the drug to be released in 2007 or 2008. Factories to produce the drug were already under construction.

In late 2006, however, reports that torcetrapib raised blood pressure in some patients emerged, and in December 2006, a research study showed a higher death rate in patients who received the new drug compared with those who received a placebo. Pfizer closed down the trial and stopped further research on the drug. The market value of Pfizer fell by about $20 billion. The news came just a few months after Bristol-Myers Squibb gave up on a potential blockbuster drug for diabetes, and Astra Zeneca halted the development of a novel medication for strokes.

There is nothing like the experience of losing billions of dollars on such gambles to focus the leadership of for-profit companies on reaping rewards when innovations *do* work out. Thus, prices of new drugs and other technologies have little to do with the cost of producing the product or the magnitude of the investment required to bring it to market. Prices are determined by what the market will bear.

When that market is the United States and the issue is life versus death, the market has been willing to bear a lot. For example, a cancer drug called Avastin was approved in 2008 for the treatment of metastatic breast cancer. The treatment costs about $92,000 a year, and its main benefit is that it delays the progression of the cancer by about five and a half months—but this drug has *not* been shown to help women with breast cancer live longer. The estimated lifetime cost of the drugs that have extended the life expectancy of patients with HIV is $618,900, or $2,100 per month [15]. Iressa costs about $1,700 per month, and a more recent drug that works in a similar way is priced even higher.

Compelling arguments have been made that the costs of medical progress is money well spent [16], but there surely is some limit to the number of $20,000 a year drugs that society can afford. The costs of less expensive interventions for healthy people also add up. For example, the number of diseases for which vaccines are widely used for children increased from seven in 1985 to fifteen for boys and sixteen for girls by 2006. With these new vaccines, the cost for the full immunization of children rose from $45 to $900 (boys) and $1,200 (girls) during this period [17].

And these are only the *direct* costs of progress and innovation. There are also *indirect* costs from medical progress, such as the higher prices of teaching hospitals, where physicians and researchers like Lynch and Haber take care of patients, do research, and make small talk that occasionally leads to breakthroughs. An operation or an MRI scan at a teaching hospital costs more than the same procedure in a freestanding facility, but the higher costs at the academic medical center help support teaching, research, and the around-the-clock availability of the latest technologies and superspecialized physicians.

There is considerable public support for academic medical centers to pursue their teaching and research missions, despite the higher costs that result. On the other hand, there is less sympathy for the other indirect costs of medical progress—the ones that result from a poorly organized health care system in which physicians are uncertain of what they should be doing as individuals, and frequently failing to coordinate their efforts with the patient or their colleagues; in short, the chaos that is so often a result of progress.

How Progress Produces Chaos

Progress is good, of course, but it generates chaos and challenges health care in at least six major ways.

1. *Too much to do*   Once a test or treatment is shown to have beneficial effects, it should be delivered to those patients who might benefit. That means physicians must screen patients and try to discern which ones are candidates, talk to the patient (and family) about the intervention, and then make sure that the patients actually get the test or treatment. These new processes must occur without any real increase in the duration of physician visits, and—all too often—without systems to help the physicians carry them out. The result: the 55 percent reliability rate described by Elizabeth McGlynn and colleagues [18].

2. *Physicians feel less competent*   As more is known, physicians feel less knowledgeable as individuals. When they do not know which test to order, they often order all of them. They refer patients to specialists for problems that were bread-and-butter issues for them just a few years ago—like the management of diabetes—because of concern that they cannot provide up-to-date care.

3. *Expanded role for specialists*   With so much to know and so many procedures to master, it takes more specialists with narrower fields of expertise to give state-of-the-art care. But the culture and organizational structure of medicine have not emphasized coordination among physicians to date.

4. *Expanded roles for nonphysicians*   When scientific progress clarifies the right thing to do, a physician is often no longer necessary to do it. Thus, a natural consequence of progress is the enlargement of the roles of nurses, pharmacists, and other nonphysician caregivers—including the patients themselves. Again, the culture and organization of medicine have not emphasized coordination among them.

5. *Multiple sites of care*   As progress advances, innovations diffuse from teaching hospitals to community hospitals and doctors' offices, and even patients' homes. Patients therefore receive their care from more people, but also at more sites. The flow of information among these people at these various sites is far from reliable.

6. *Patients are more demanding*   A demanding generation (the baby boomers) and a media inclined to meet its needs yields a patient population highly interested in receiving the most recent innovations, even when older and less expensive treatments and tests are reasonable. Many of these patients are insistent on preserving their freedom to choose whichever physician or hospital might give them the best care—even if they have difficulty knowing which ones are actually best, and even though moving among provider organizations increases the likelihood of failures in communication.

The chaos that results from these indirect effects of progress is expensive and infuriating. And it can be overcome. But doing so requires understanding how twenty-first-century medical knowledge imposed on a twentieth-century delivery system is a prescription for failure. The next chapter will examine in greater detail the ways in which our knowledge of how to deliver care has not kept up with our knowledge of what we can and should do.

3   Fragmentation

The conventional wisdom is that the U.S. health care system is broken, but that assessment is misleading. After all, can a system that has never truly existed be called broken? All of the components of fabulous health care exist in abundance in the United States, yet with a few exceptions, they have never been organized to work together. These health care providers are small and not-so-small businesses performing their specific roles—virtually all of which are altruistic and honorable. But these providers have not yet been asked, encouraged, cajoled, or forced to work together around the common goal of meeting a population's health care needs.

The phrase "The U.S. health care system is broken" logically leads to the follow-up question "Who broke it?" As we have argued in the earlier chapters, our assessment is that villains are not to blame for our challenges; the real problem is that recent progress has unmasked the chaos that results from the lack of a provider organization. A more useful assessment is "U.S. health care is fragmented," and the right follow-up question is "How do we organize those pieces into a system that can use its components to meet patients' needs?" Our optimistic assessment is that U.S. health care has not failed; it is just getting down to the work of meeting the needs of our times—and not a moment too soon.

Even with minimal organization, there are many instances in every city every day in which U.S. health care performs brilliantly. Critical illnesses are immediately diagnosed, and patients are quickly transferred to settings in which they can receive treatment from experienced clinicians. People with increased risks for chronic diseases like diabetes and hypertension receive education on how to improve their outlook. Patients who have had heart attacks routinely receive medications that reduce their death rate.

In the absence of true organization into delivery systems, however, providers often do not communicate with each other or coordinate their efforts. Most U.S. physicians work in small, one or two doctor practices, with paper medical records that are inaccessible to their colleagues, hospitals, and patients. Hospitals, doctors, nursing homes, and home care agencies are separate entities that cooperate on some issues but compete on others. Multiple insurers supply a patchwork system of coverage, each using their own administrative systems, adding complexity and costs.

This fragmentation is not limited to the components of our health care system; it also characterizes the way in which patients and their illnesses are viewed. To cope with the flood of scientific knowledge described in chapter 2, physicians are divided into increasingly narrow subspecialties defined by organs and diseases. Health insurers pay providers on the basis of individual physician office visits, hospitalizations, tests, and procedures—not the episodes of weeks, months, and years that actually define an illness. Some medical conditions, particularly mental illness, are "carved out" from the rest of health care by some insurance companies, and handled completely separately by different payment systems and different networks of doctors.

This fragmentation is familiar to patients who feel that the health care system has forgotten that they are people, not just diseases. And it poses a fundamental barrier to addressing problems that demand complex solutions, such as an aging population in which many patients have multiple conditions that require numerous medications and numerous physicians and nonphysicians, often located in multiple institutions. The fragmentation also complicates the task of meeting the desires for information from an increasingly busy and sophisticated population that is accustomed to getting what it wants 24–7.

These challenges grow more pressing each year owing to scientific progress that produces new tests and treatments. The good news is that we know more than ever about what to do, but the bad news is that our knowledge of how to do it lags far behind. Put another way, our scientific knowledge is expanding at a much faster rate than our expertise in how to deliver health care that is timely, safe, reliable, and efficient.

Indeed, the mismatch between medical knowledge and our ability to manage it has reached a point where the status quo is unsustainable—and change actually is under way. In this chapter, we complete our description of the context for that change, which is the chaos that results from rapid progress imposed on a fragmented health care delivery system.

The Nonsystem

The fragmentation of U.S. health care was not an obvious problem before the recent explosion of knowledge from medical research. A generation ago, there were fewer tests, which provided much less information; fewer medications, many of which did not actually work; and fewer operations, which entailed more risk and more pain. In that era, medicine was more talk and less action, because there just weren't that many treatments that helped patients get better. Physicians earned respect and loyalty by hovering by the bedside of the critically ill. Wise teachers told medical students, "Don't just do something; stand there." We didn't need the phrase of "primary care physician" because your doctor was usually your only doctor. There was less risk for miscommunication, and less danger from drug interactions and other inadvertent injuries—the medical equivalent of friendly fire.

Everyone waxes nostalgic for those days, when life was simpler, relationships were deeper, and costs were lower. But would anyone really trade the medicine of today for the less expensive health care available thirty years ago? Would anyone turn the clock back to a time when little could be done to prevent heart attack and stroke, or detect cancers when they were still curable?

Nevertheless, what conclusions can we draw from data showing that in a single year, the typical Medicare enrollee sees seven different physicians [1]? These seven physicians include two different primary care physicians and five specialists who collectively worked in four different practices. The number of different physicians is even higher for patients with diabetes, coronary artery disease, lung cancer, and other medical conditions (table 3.1). Keep in mind as you examine table 3.1 that these different practices probably use paper records that are not easily accessible outside their walls (and may not be legible to colleagues even within the same practice).

Why would patients see more than one primary care physician? In many cases, patients needed care when their primary care physician was unavailable (weekends, vacations, etc.). But about 20 percent of patients changed their primary care physicians during the period of 2000 to 2002, and there was even greater movement of patients among

Table 3.1
Number of physicians who treated Medicare beneficiaries in 2000

Patient group (by condition)	Number of unique providers (median)			
	Total physicians	Primary care physicians	Specialists	Practices
All	7	2	5	4
Diabetes	8	3	6	5
Coronary artery disease	10	3	7	6
Lung cancer	11	3	8	6

physicians outside of primary care. The result is that most patients receive only a minority of their care from any given physician or practice in any given year, and most doctors do not have a stable population of patients for whom they feel totally responsible.

An important consequence of this lack of organization of health care is tremendous variation in practice patterns. This variation is apparent on a national scale, with Medicare spending per beneficiary ranging from $5,200 in some regions to about $14,000 in others—without any evidence of better health outcomes for Medicare patients in the higher cost regions [2, 3]. About 40 percent of this variation can be explained by differences in prices and the illnesses of the underlying populations, but about 60 percent seems to be due to other factors, such as the supply of medical resources (doctors, hospital beds, and radiology testing equipment) and local practice norms [4].

In truth, though, local practice norms hardly exist in a fragmented health care system. In our own organization in Boston, two- to three-fold variation in the use of various tests often exists among physicians at the same hospital in the same specialty. In most cases, those physicians who order more tests than their colleagues and those who order fewer are unaware that they differ in their practice patterns from colleagues who are literally down the hall.

A Fragmented Approach to Payment

Why are physicians unaware of the variation in their practice patterns within their own community? For most, the payment system has not provided a compelling reason for them to think of themselves as anything more than individual physicians trying to do a good job for the individual patients in front of them. That payment system has not

Table 3.2
How the payment system is fragmented

---

1. Failure to cover everyone
2. Multiple payers with multiple incentive and payment systems
3. Fee-for-service payment structure that compensates providers for individual units of service
4. Providers not directly rewarded for meeting patients' long-term needs
5. Often no penalty for doing the wrong thing
6. Payers' relationships with patients are short term
7. Patients largely insulated from costs of health care
8. Mental health carved out from rest of health care by some health plans
9. No one has all the information
10. No one has all the responsibility

---

posed the question of whether groups of doctors might deliver better care by coordinating their work and comparing their practice patterns to those of one another.

Thus, the fragmentation of U.S. health care is reflected in and sustained by the way it is financed. Our payment system evolved during the last century, when employers were competing for workers, the overall costs of health care were much lower, and little was known about how to prevent premature death. The goal was to provide protection from financial ruin when medical catastrophe occurred.

No wonder, then, that this payment system is not up to the challenges of our times. Table 3.2 portrays our summary of the ways in which the U.S. payment system breaks up the delivery of health care or breaks down itself in the effort to meet the long-term needs of Americans.

The most glaring gap is the lack of a national insurance system that guarantees a basic level of care to every citizen—a social commitment made by every other developed country (and many not-so-developed ones). Instead, the United States has a patchwork system with multiple public and private payers, each with its own policies, incentive programs, and claims payment systems. Each of these payment systems requires the development of a corresponding set of policies and procedures in hospitals and physician practices.

Much has been made of these administrative costs and the holes in this patchwork system through which about 47 million Americans fall without insurance. These are huge issues that are not to be taken lightly. But there are more subtle problems in our payment systems that may be as important—problems that could be addressed without a complete upheaval of our multipayer system.

Among these basic problems are what we pay for, and what we do *not* pay for. We generally do not pay for keeping people healthy or even for making them better. Instead, we break down the relationships between patients and health care providers into bite-size interactions—individual units of service like office visits, days in the hospital, tests, and procedures.

In health care like any other activity in which money changes hands, you tend to get what you pay for. If you pay for office visits, you get more office visits. If you pay for tests and operations, you get more of those as well. We are not implying that our colleagues spend their days milking the system financially and doing things to patients solely to generate income. There are sociopaths in health care who do just that, of course, but our experience suggests that they are the rare exception, not the rule.

Still, to do well under the current payment system, physicians and hospitals must provide services for which the compensation exceeds the costs. And to ensure adequate time and resources for their work, they tend to restrict the percentage of their activities that are uncompensated or are not profitable.

Even nonprofit organizations committed to helping the poor have to pay their personnel competitively or risk losing them. To do so, they try to increase their volumes of profitable services like surgical operations and radiology tests, while containing growth in activities like mental health and primary care, for which the compensation may not cover the costs. At for-profit organizations dominated by the commitment to increase shareholder value, the focus on profitable activities is even stronger [5].

The problem, then, is what is not paid for—or what is not compensated sufficiently well to make it profitable. Physicians who are paid by the visit are not rewarded for investing in systems designed to improve patients' long-term health, like computer systems that keep track of diabetic patients. Hospitals have no direct incentive to implement programs that prevent hospital admissions for patients with heart failure or other chronic diseases.

Just as the payment system does not reward some activities that are beneficial to patients, it also does not provide much punishment when the *wrong* thing happens. When complications occur to patients, clinicians feel horrible, of course. But there is usually no direct financial penalty; in fact, the prolonged hospitalizations as well as additional tests and treatments may mean *more* revenue to hospitals and doctors.

How can such a shortsighted payment system endure? One reason is that the relationships between the organizations paying for health care (employers and insurance companies) and patients are often transitory. People change employers, and employers change health plans frequently, so neither insurers nor employers can assume that they will have any particular member for more than a year or two.

Short time horizons discourage investments like hypertension control or weight loss programs, in which cost savings might be realized years later. Instead of funding a health care system designed to improve and protect health, insurance tends to focus on two other functions. The first is catastrophic protection—that is, the coverage of health care costs if a patient has a major illness. And the second is group purchasing—that is, holding down prices on the units of service that they are "buying" for patients' routine health care needs, such as physician office visits and hospital rates. Employers and insurers are not happy with this approach, but they often do not have other options.

Even when employers are responsible for the long-term health care costs of their employees and retirees, they approach their commitments in a businesslike way. For example, we and our colleagues at Partners HealthCare System once proposed developing a heart failure program for a large employer's population of retirees. Heart failure programs have been proven to help people with this condition live longer, feel better, and stay out of the hospital. The employer responded that the concept was appealing, but the main financial benefit of the program would be decreased hospitalizations, which were covered for the retirees by Medicare. Hence, the federal government would enjoy savings from our heart failure program, rather than the employer whom we were asking to fund the program. The employer expressed embarrassment and regret, but declined our proposal without hesitation.

We never discussed asking patients with heart failure to pay for that program, even though many of them might have been willing to do so if they understood its potential benefits. We did not ask because U.S. patients have traditionally been insulated from the costs of their care—a type of fragmentation that has an obvious appeal to patients and their doctors, neither of whom want financial concerns to have undue influence in life-and-death decisions. Most decisions in medicine are not life and death, however, and when neither physician nor patient has reason to hesitate before using an expensive intervention, the risk of the inefficient use of resources is obvious.

Frustrated by their inability to control costs through their interactions with patients or physicians, many insurance companies have taken a divide-and-conquer approach. Some insurers separate psychiatric disease from the rest of medical care, and allow patients to go only to a small subset of mental health clinicians who have agreed to take low payment rates and adhere to rigid management protocols. These carve outs help the insurance company hold down costs, but splinter patients' care, so that primary care physicians often do not even know the names of the psychiatrists or psychologists seeing their patients, or what drugs have been prescribed by them. On a superficial level, mental health carve outs provide some financial predictability to insurance companies unnerved by the potentially limitless appetite of people for psychiatric therapy. Yet does it really make sense to handle schizophrenia differently from Parkinson's disease, when both are diseases of the brain with a known biochemical basis?

Payers and employers frequently extend this divide-and-conquer approach to their negotiations with health care providers. Many purchasers would rather discuss fees and rates with fragmented providers, who have little negotiating power, than sit across the contracting table from a larger organization that might be able to offer more coordinated care but also has a stronger negotiating position.

But in the fragmented health care world that results, no one has all the information of what is going on with a given patient, and no one assumes the responsibility to ensure that everything that should be done gets done and that mistakes are not made. The consequence is that the payers add work-arounds and layers to the health care system, such as disease management companies that hire nurses to call and check on high-risk patients, and that sift through claims looking for patients who have not had tests that they need. Pharmacy benefit management companies examine prescriptions that might be changed to a more cost-effective medication. All this extra activity does help some patients, but it adds to the costs and chaos of U.S. health care today.

In this environment, it is not easy for a provider organization to take a broad perspective and design its care to optimize patients' interests *and* efficiency. But just as flowers push their way up through cracks in concrete, good things sometimes happen despite opposing business incentives. The redesign of care for patients with back pain by physicians at Virginia Mason Medical Center is such a story. This example, however, also shows the obstacles that can prevent such flowers from flourishing.

Virginia Mason Medical Center is an integrated provider organization with 480 physicians and a 300-bed hospital in downtown Seattle, Washington, along with ambulatory surgical care centers and outpatient facilities throughout the region. (More detail on this organization will be provided in chapter 5.) In 2004, leaders of Virginia Mason began working with a national insurer (Aetna) and major local employers such as Starbucks to help address rising costs for common problems, including low back pain. They ultimately created a system in which patients with low back pain are triaged immediately to physical therapists—the one intervention for back pain that has actually been shown to help patients recover. By sending patients directly to physical therapy, Virginia Mason reduced their need for appointments with primary care physicians and specialists, and high-cost radiology tests like CT scans and MRIs. The patients get better faster, with much less waiting, and at a lower cost.

Everyone wins, right? Well not quite. It turns out that CT and MRI scans are profitable for Virginia Mason, while physical therapy is a money loser. The redesigned back pain approach cuts out the not-so-useful tests that subsidize the treatment that actually works. To try to correct the perverse incentives, Aetna and the employers negotiated a new contract that pays Virginia Mason more for physical therapy if it can reach a targeted 50 percent reduction in low back MRI.

At first glance, this might seem a happy ending to the story. But will it really make sense for Virginia Mason to push physical therapy as the first line of treatment for patients with back pain if other insurers do not also change their payment strategies? After all, Aetna only covers about 10 percent of the market in Seattle, so it wouldn't be wise for Virginia Mason to maintain an approach that is profitable for Aetna patients, but loses money for all its other patients. For this program to survive and spread, insurers have to move beyond paying for tests and figure out how to pay for care.

A Fragmented Provider System

Even if the insurance plans in the U.S. health care system were ready to pay for well-coordinated care for populations of patients, they would not find many health care providers able to meet the challenge (table 3.3). A major reason is that most U.S. physicians work alone or close to

Table 3.3
How the provider system is fragmented

1. Predominance of one or two physician practices
2. Primary care physicians delivering smaller portion of care
3. Silos among specialties
4. Lack of collaboration between physicians and hospitals
5. Lack of shared information systems
6. Reliance on individual physician responsibility for protection of quality

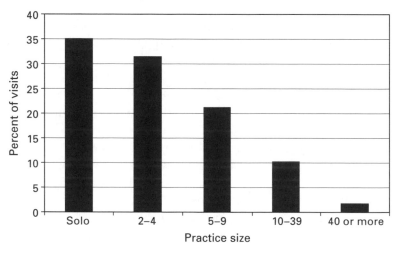
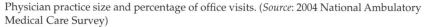

Figure 3.1
Physician practice size and percentage of office visits. (*Source*: 2004 National Ambulatory Medical Care Survey)

it. Health care is delivered predominantly by physicians who own or co-own their medical practices, and most of those practices are small and do not have electronic systems that allow for reliable communication with other physicians. In a country that celebrates rugged individualism, U.S. doctors are only slowly adapting to the concept of modern medicine as a team sport.

The extent to which health care is splintered is captured in data from the 2004 National Ambulatory Medical Care Survey [6], which found that 87 percent of all office visits were to physicians who owned the practice themselves or with other physicians. More than one-third of the visits were to physicians who practiced alone. Two-thirds of the visits were to groups smaller than five physicians (figure 3.1). Care

provided by large groups of physicians employed by a health maintenance organization or an academic medical center was the exception,
not the rule.

More than half of these visits were to specialists—a reflection of the
growing proportion of health care being delivered by specialists. That
increase is driven by medical advances that require knowledge and
experience acquired during years of training in a specialty. But the
flip side of that coin is that primary care physicians are doing less
and less.

How dramatic is this trend? In 2004, researchers released the results
of a survey of twenty-five hundred general internists who were
members of the American College of Physicians, a prestigious professional society [7]. In this study, the physicians were asked which
common medical procedures they had performed during the last year
(table 3.4). When these data were compared to results from a similar
1986 survey, the researchers found that the percentage of general internists doing each procedure had fallen by about half.

The findings suggest that primary care physicians have become
uncomfortable doing medical procedures that were routine for their
predecessors from a generation before. The treadmill exercise tests are
now being done by the cardiologists, the lumbar punctures are being
done by the neurologists, and so on. This trend is not limited to primary
care physicians; even among specialists, subsets of them who focus on
performing the procedures are emerging. One new term that has just
begun to emerge at many hospitals is "proceduralist," to describe physicians whose sole role is to perform certain medical procedures such

Table 3.4
Percentage of general internists reporting that they had done specific medical procedures
in prior year

Procedure	1986	2004
Treadmill exercise test	45%	29%
Lumbar puncture (spinal tap)	73%	26%
Thoracentesis (drainage of fluid from chest)	66%	23%
Endotracheal tube placement	41%	15%
Elective cardioversion (using electric shock to correct abnormal heart rhythm)	38%	8%
Bone marrow aspiration	37%	8%
Liver biopsy	17%	2%

as the insertion of large intravenous lines. The sought-after result is better technical skill, but the price paid is the loss of a relationship between the patient and the physician performing the procedure.

Even though primary care physicians call for help from specialists more often now, *most* of the specialist visits captured in the 2004 National Ambulatory Care Survey were *not* initiated by a referral from another physician. Patients apparently went to the specialists on their own, so there presumably were no primary care physicians expecting to receive the specialists' reports. Even when there *is* a primary care physician, however, communication breakdowns with specialists are all too common.

Communication failures are common not just among physicians in outpatient settings but also between clinicians at different sites of care [8]. These breakdowns are particularly common—and risky—when patients are discharged from the hospital. These patients are, of course, the sickest and most fragile, and need to be seen by their outpatient physicians shortly after discharge. These physicians need to know what tests were performed as well as what drugs were started and stopped during the admission. The usual way to pass on such information is a discharge summary that is dictated by one of the hospital-based doctors, and then mailed, faxed, or emailed to the primary care physician.

A recent review of published data shows how rarely the system works the way one would hope [9]. Researchers found that discharge summaries were available at the first postdischarge office visit only 12 to 34 percent of the time. Even four weeks after a discharge, discharge summaries were available to primary care physicians just 51 to 77 percent of the time. The quality of care was compromised in 25 percent of follow-up visits.

These failures in communication are not surprising when one considers that only rarely are physicians part of the same business entity as the hospitals to which they admit patients. Physicians are usually the owners of their own small businesses, and they in fact often have testy relationships with their hospitals over various financial issues (e.g., whether physicians provide highly profitable laboratory services, thereby reducing hospitals' sources of profit that might be needed to subsidize other hospital functions) [10, 11]. The ability of hospitals and physicians to cooperate on the flow of information and overall coordination of patients' care is highly variable, and currently questionable in many communities.

Patients can reduce the risk of faulty communication if they carry the information to the outpatient physicians themselves on paper or via a computerized personal health record, or if they only see physicians within a single organization using a single EMR. Yet patients tend to resist any restrictions on which physicians they can see. They fear that they will not be able to see the best physicians when they need to; they want to be able to go anywhere to see any doctor. What is the trade-off for this freedom of choice? Their physicians frequently have to work with only part of the information they need.

In an age when Apple computers can talk to Windows machines, one would think that patients should be able to go to physicians anywhere, and that their EMRs should be able to communicate with each other. And someday we will likely get there. For now, however, most physicians are *not* using electronic records, and the available electronic records cannot transmit information to other systems except through clunky means like emails with attachments that are copied into the receiving doctor's information system.

The U.S. public is surprised that these information systems cannot communicate with each other, but unwittingly preserves this fragmentation by opposing the concept of a universal patient identification number (UPIN). UPINs would allow information systems to identify individuals reliably and then integrate their clinical data. But many Americans believe that a UPIN would make identity theft easier or otherwise threaten the confidentiality of their medical data. Thus, physicians must use email to send data to colleagues in other organizations, review each piece of information to be sure they are talking about the right patient, and then copy the data into the record.

Concern that the confidentiality of medical information might be threatened by computerization is certainly valid. Hackers try to invade the information systems of hospitals and other health care providers on a daily basis. And patients fear that knowledge of their medical issues (e.g., HIV infection or diabetes) could adversely affect their personal and work relationships, or their ability to get insurance.

Nevertheless, the availability of information to patients' clinicians at any time and place can be lifesaving. In addition, security systems for electronic data are good and getting better. We can identify every individual who has accessed a patient's electronic record, but we cannot tell who has opened a patient's paper record. The irony is that if we all had UPINs, information could be shared more safely electronically and confidentiality would be more secure. On this issue, concerns about confidentiality have the potential to reinforce the fragmentation of care and compromise quality.

A Cultural Revolution Begins

Like their patients, doctors suffer from the disorganization and fragmentation of the health care system. They spend too much time in frustrating searches for information that they need, and go home too many evenings wondering if a critical issue is slipping through the cracks. Why do they tolerate the chaos?

It is not easy to give up the culture in which one was raised, and most physicians in leadership roles today were trained in an era in which the quality of care depended almost completely on individual responsibility. A generation ago, there were few, if any, data by which to evaluate care. Medical records on patients were illegible and scattered in the offices of their physicians (i.e., the cardiologist had the cardiology information, the oncologist had the cancer-related information, and no one had all the information).

Even if all the data had been accessible, it would still have been difficult to evaluate quality of care for a simple reason: there was much less clarity on what the right thing to do might be. Rigorously performed clinical trials only became commonplace in medicine in the last few decades. Prior to that, there were few research studies that compared new drugs with a placebo or one test against another. Today, the term "evidence-based medicine" is a standard for excellence, describing an approach to patient care in which physicians use data from research studies to guide their care. But the phrase itself was introduced for the first time in 1992 [12].

An awkward but obvious question is, What were physicians basing their decisions on before they started using evidence? Like apprentices training in a craft, they learned by emulating their teachers. They shared anecdotes and were heavily influenced by what had happened to the last patient they had seen with a similar problem. They relied on their instincts.

The nature of medicine made it hard to tell who was doing a good job and who was not. When bad things happened to patients, there were logical explanations—after all, they were sick, frail, and often old. And because the human body is remarkably resilient, the vast majority of mistakes made by physicians did not actually cause detectable harm. In the prescientific era of medicine, physicians were respected for working so hard on behalf of their patients and were given the benefit of the doubt.

Medicine at present is more science than craft, though, and the heroic lone healer is fast becoming an anachronism. At least some dimensions of the quality of care provided by individual physicians *can* be measured now, and "report cards" for many physicians are readily available on the Internet. When data are used to rank physicians, there are three possible outcomes: they can come out above average, average, or below average. Since no patients like to think of their physicians as mediocre, two out these three outcomes are bad from the perspective of the doctor.

If these report cards threaten the heroic image of physicians, medical progress itself has made the lone aspect of doctoring impossible. No one can deliver modern state-of-the-art care to complex, sick patients on their own anymore. Physicians need to work in teams with other clinicians, including nonphysician colleagues such as nurses and pharmacists. Teams need a playbook so everyone knows what they are supposed to do. And they need ways of communicating so that everyone knows what is happening.

Working in teams does not come easily to physicians whose self-image is akin to that of Charles Lindbergh—the Lone Eagle. They treasure their autonomy, and some still scorn guidelines as "cookbook medicine." They mourn the days when no decision was made without their knowledge and consent, and many say that they would never have gone into medicine if they knew what it was going to be like today.

Revolutions occur when older paradigms become unsustainable, and scientific progress is having just that effect on the fragmented version of the U.S. health care system. Payers, providers, and patients are all looking for new ways to finance health care [13]. And they know that the delivery of the care itself must change dramatically, too.

As traumatic as the changes may be for older physicians trained in another era, a new generation of physicians is on the way. They are computer savvy. They are not trained to believe that they should know everything; instead, they learn how to find out what they need to know and how to work in teams. The shape of an organized health system is beginning to emerge.

II The Solution Is Organization

4   What Does Organization in Health Care Look Like?

Most Americans know what disorganized health care is like. Amid a swirl of activity in our hospitals and physician offices, patients wait—for appointments, test results, and clear information that sometimes never comes. Physicians cannot reach each other, and thus do not give patients consistent or coherent answers to questions. Tests are duplicated by accident or forgotten altogether. Abnormal test results are overlooked. Costs are high, and quality is disappointing.

Patients and providers who have known nothing but disorganized care have been accepting of this chaos, but medical progress is intensifying the cost and quality problems that result. Providers *and* purchasers are beginning to recognize the powerful forces that tend to fragment health care, and understand that serious efforts to counter that fragmentation are necessary. Indeed, some policy experts now argue that there is an inherent "goodness to groupness," because organized groups of providers can take responsibility for issues that individual physicians cannot—issues such as care for the uninsured, conflicts of interest, and responsibility for a population of patients over time.

The very concept that health care *can* be organized is still new in many circles, but the evidence is accumulating that organized providers can adopt systems beyond the reach of disorganized providers. Several studies have shown that larger physician groups and physicians who are members in networks are more likely to use EMRs, have quality improvement programs, and deliver higher-quality care than small groups or solo physician practices [1–4]. Small hospitals that are owned by multihospital systems have more advanced information technology systems than independent hospitals of similar size [5]. Some data indicate that the greater the degree of organization of providers, the higher the quality [6–8].

From data such as these, the ingredients for major improvement through the organization of health care are emerging. In this chapter, we will give a broad overview of the themes that characterize organized health care. We begin with an optimistic perspective on what is possible, based on a recent example in which the entire U.S. health care system became highly reliable with regard to one important quality issue. The overall picture is not as sterling as this one example would suggest, of course, and we compare the U.S. health care system with some real-life benchmarks that reflect organization and coordination. Then, we turn to the specific features that define organized health care, and consider what they imply for several different types of patients.

Progress Is Possible: A National Success Story

On May 8, 2007, one of the best-known quality measures in health care was retired, and for the best of reasons: it was no longer useful. Since 1996, the National Committee for Quality Assurance (NCQA) had been evaluating U.S. HMOs on the percentage of patients with acute myocardial infarction who receive a prescription for beta-blockers within seven days after a hospital discharge. But in 2007, the NCQA stopped asking HMOs to keep track of this performance measure.

This news was surprising at first glance, because beta-blockers are a class of medications that greatly reduce the risk of death for patients who have had heart attacks. Despite many research studies showing their benefit, only about half of heart attack patients received this therapy as recently as the mid-1990s. By 2005, however, almost all heart attack survivors received beta-blockers, and the difference between the ninetieth and the tenth percentile of HMOs—the best and the worst—had shrunk to a few percentage points [9] (figure 4.1). On this issue at least, the entire U.S. health care system had become reliable.

How did such dramatic improvement occur over the course of a decade? The real success story actually took considerably longer. It began on March 26, 1982, with the publication of the Beta-Blocker Heart Attack Trial (BHAT) in the *Journal of the American Medical Association* [10]. BHAT was a large study sponsored by the National Institutes of Health in which patients who had had heart attacks were randomly assigned to receive a medication named propranolol or a placebo that was identical in appearance.

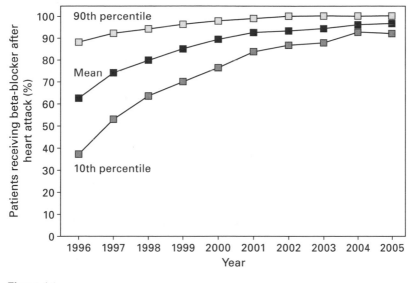

Figure 4.1
Use of beta-blocker treatment after myocardial infarction, 1996–2005. (Reproduced with permission from the *New England Journal of Medicine* 2007;357:1175–1177)

Propranolol is one of the oldest beta-blockers, a class of drugs that blocks the effects of adrenaline and slows the heart down. (Other widely used beta-blockers include atenolol, metoprolol, and nadolol.) Until BHAT, the conventional wisdom was that beta-blockers were too dangerous to give to patients who had had heart attacks because they might weaken an already-damaged heart. In fact, when the authors were young physicians in training, we were taught *never* to give beta-blockers to patients who had had heart attacks. During the 1970s, however, research on animals in laboratories suggested that beta-blockers might actually protect the heart from further injury. Small pilot studies in humans provided further encouragement, so the National Institutes of Health invested millions of dollars to enroll 3,837 patients in BHAT to determine whether the benefits of beta-blockers might exceed their risks.

Few were prepared for just how wrong the conventional wisdom turned out to be. The researchers actually stopped the BHAT study nine months early because patients who received propranolol were doing so much better than the placebo group. Subsequent data indicate that beta-blockers cut the death rate after heart attacks by as much as 40 percent.

Another pleasant surprise was that patients in whom beta-blockers had been avoided in the past also benefit from these drugs after heart attacks. As expected, patients with chronic obstructive pulmonary disease (emphysema), heart failure, and advanced age had a greater risk of side effects from beta-blockers, but they also had a greater risk of dying from their heart attacks—so they turned out to be *more* likely to benefit from beta-blockers than other heart attack patients. The bottom line was that the benefits of beta-blockers exceeded the risks even for the very patients most likely to have side effects [11]. Instead of stopping or withholding beta-blockers, as was the established practice, physicians should have been giving them routinely to virtually every heart attack patient.

In an ideal world, after landmark studies like BHAT, doctors would change their treatment patterns within a few weeks. But the painful reality is that such change is usually slow and incomplete, even when the findings are dramatic and the disease is life threatening. A major study, for example, that proved the benefits of aspirin for patients with heart attacks was published in 1988. Over the next three years, the use of aspirin in such patients increased from 39 percent to just 72 percent [12]—real progress, to be sure, but not impressive if you happened to be one of the 28 percent of the heart attack patients who did not get aspirin in 1991. (Today, close to 100 percent of patients with heart attacks receive aspirin.)

If good research is necessary but not sufficient to drive sweeping change, what are the other key ingredients? How do you persuade doctors that something they were admonished *never* to do should now be done on every patient? The next step is acceptance by key opinion leaders, with such opinions first expressed in editorials and review articles in leading medical journals, and then in textbooks. In the case of beta-blockers after heart attacks, that acceptance came quickly. By 1984, the benefits of beta-blockers for heart attack patients were cited in the second edition of the bible of modern cardiology, Eugene Braunwald's *Heart Disease* [13].

The endorsement of experts helps, but it is not enough to drive change all the way through the health care system—and by the mid-1990s, the percentage of patients with heart attacks who received beta-blockers was still just 34 percent in one major study [11] and 38 percent in another [14]. Around that time, though, experts were beginning to find a powerful new way to express their opinions: through guidelines that offered specific recommendations for well-defined subsets of patients. In 1996, the American College of Cardiology and the American Heart Association published recommendations for heart attack care that included the use of beta-blockers.

With the availability of that consensus of experts, organizations in the emerging field of quality measurement jumped into action. In 1997, the organization that evaluates U.S. hospitals, the Joint Commission on Accreditation of Healthcare Organizations, started a hospital-performance measurement program that included the use of beta-blockers at discharge for patients with heart attacks. The Health Care Financing Administration began collecting data on Medicare patients with heart attacks who received these drugs. And the NCQA began comparing HMOs on this new measure of quality.

Doing well on the NCQA's quality report card is a business imperative for HMOs, because their scores are used to determine whether they get NCQA accreditation—the "seal of approval" for managed care organizations. NCQA accreditation ensures that insurance companies balance the need to control costs with the needs to measure and improve quality. Many employers will not allow their employees to sign up for health care coverage through plans that do not have NCQA accreditation.

So the health plans responded to this new measure of their quality in a businesslike way. They integrated the recommendations for beta-blockers into the "scripts" used by case managers who interviewed patients who had had heart attacks, and sent those patients letters with information on beta-blockers and other risk-reducing interventions. They also sent reminder letters to physicians if claims data indicated that a patient had not received beta-blockers after a heart attack.

In the early 2000s, some health plans began offering financial incentives to hospitals to improve the reliability with which heart attack patients received beta-blockers as well as other key medical treatments that have been shown to be beneficial. Hospitals respond to the public reporting of data on their quality, but they respond even *more* when they also have such "pay-for-performance" incentives [15].

Meanwhile, professional societies began to move beyond publishing guidelines and started leading quality improvement initiatives. The American College of Cardiology had launched a program called Guidelines Applied in Practice in 1981, but the changing environment gave

Table 4.1
Key steps in performance improvement

1. Rigorous research, ideally including randomized trials
2. Acceptance of findings by opinion leaders
3. Development of guidelines
4. Development of performance measures based on guidelines
5. Use of performance measures in:
a. Internal quality improvement programs
b. Public report cards
c. Pay-for-performance contracts between payers and providers
6. Development of quality improvement collaboratives to share best practices
7. Implementation of systems that ensure reliable delivery of the appropriate medical intervention

the program new energy [16]. The other leading cardiovascular disease society, the American Heart Association, started its own initiative for hospital improvement, Get with the Guidelines [17]. Additional momentum was provided by the Institute for Healthcare Improvement's 100,000 Lives Campaign and its successor, the 5 Million Lives Campaign, both of which included beta-blocker treatment after heart attacks as one of their priorities [18].

A few years into the new century, it was clear that virtually all U.S. patients with heart attacks were getting at least a trial of beta-blockers. It had taken twenty-five years for the findings in BHAT to exert their full influence. But this experience and others have helped define the key steps needed to achieve highly reliable health care (see table 4.1).

There is good reason to believe that the next BHAT will take much less than a quarter century to cause sweeping change in care. The development and updating of guidelines is now a well-practiced business for professional societies like the American College of Cardiology and the American Heart Association. National, state, and local organizations are developing quality measures, and reporting on how hospitals and doctors perform. Quality improvement collaboratives were a foreign concept a decade ago, but are now emerging as ongoing regional efforts in many parts of the country.

At the risk of seeming overly optimistic, we are willing to argue that U.S. health care is learning how to learn. We have improved our very ability to improve. But now let's turn back to reality, and confront the gap between what is and what could be.

How Organized Are We? A Report Card

In 2006, the Commonwealth Fund Commission on a High Performance Health System (which was chaired by one of us, JJM) published a national scorecard on U.S. health care [19]. As noted in chapter 1, this commission did not compare U.S. health care against perfection but instead used real performance data, usually from the top 10 percent of countries, states, health plans, hospitals, or other providers. If the best real-life performance for some measure of quality was 80 percent, and the United States averaged 40 percent, for example, then the score for the United States would be fifty for that measure.

The initial report card made headlines in 2006 because of the mediocre overall performance that it described for the U.S. health care system, and the scores were no better in 2008 when an update was released [20]. In 2008, the overall score for all thirty-seven measures was sixty-five (slightly worse than the sixty-six score from 2006), with scores ranging from thirty-five for efficiency to ninety for quality. Some of these measures are strongly influenced by the overall health of Americans—such as the overall death rate. On the other hand, several of the measures are direct reflections of the degree of organization of U.S. health care. Key measures and the scores for the country overall that are related to the organization of care are summarized in table 4.2.

Collectively, the disappointing scores on these measures help describe what is missing from U.S. health care. The problems are not due to physicians who are not smart enough or do not work hard enough. Rather, the problems are due to the inability to coordinate the care of individual patients among multiple providers, keep track of populations of patients over time, and engage patients themselves in their own care. For a substantial subset of the thirty-seven measures, the fundamental challenge is not finding the money to pay for the care we deliver. The challenge instead is organizing patients and clinicians to make that care better.

Aims and Visions for Organized Health Care

Now let's move closer to the ground level of health care and consider what exactly defines well-organized health care. We need a clear idea of what greater organization means for hospitals, doctors, and patients themselves. In its famous 2001 report, *Crossing the Quality Chasm* [21],

Table 4.2
2008 national scorecard: Selected items

Indicator	Score (100 = benchmark)
Adults received recommended screening and preventive care	62
Children received recommended immunizations and preventive care	86
Needed mental health care and received treatment	76
Chronic disease under control	76
Hospitalized patients received recommended care for heart attacks, heart failure, and pneumonia	90
Adults under sixty-five with accessible primary care provider	76
Care coordination at hospital discharge	74
Patients reported medical, medication, or lab test error	59
Ability to see doctor on same/next day when sick or needed medical attention	57
Very/somewhat easy to get care after hours without going to the emergency room	35
Doctor-patient communication: always listened, explained, showed respect, and spent enough time	75
Adults with chronic conditions given self-management plan	89
Patient-centered hospital care	87
Potential overuse or waste	41
Went to emergency room for condition that could have been treated by regular doctor	29
Hospital admissions for medical conditions for which excellent outpatient care can often prevent need for hospitalization	56
Medicare hospital thirty-day readmission rates	76
Physicians using electronic medical records	29

the Institute of Medicine described six key aims for the improvement of health care:

1. *Safe*   The avoidance of injury and harm from care that is supposed to help patients

2. *Effective*   The reliable matching of "evidence-based" care to actual care; that is, providing services based on scientific knowledge to all who could benefit, and refraining from offering services to those not likely to benefit

3. *Patient centered*   The provision of care that is respectful of and responsive to individual patient preferences, needs, and values, thereby ensuring that patient values guide all clinical decisions

4. *Timely* The avoidance of unnecessary delays

5. *Efficient* The avoidance of waste, including waste of equipment, supplies, ideas, energy, and time

6. *Equitable* The provision of care that does not vary in quality because of personal characteristics such as gender, ethnicity, geographic location, and socioeconomic status

The translation of these high-level aims into specific functions for providers starts to define what success and failure mean in organized health care. A straightforward test is whether the providers can assume responsibility for the care of a population of people over time. This responsibility means doing more than offering superb care to the person sitting in front of physicians.

Organized care means ensuring that patients' key information is available when it is needed by clinicians as well as the patients themselves—a function that requires the implementation of an EMR. It means coordinating care among multiple providers who are often at multiple institutions—a function that requires both software such as EMRs, and "humanware" such as care coordination and disease management programs. And it means having the ability to measure the performance (efficiency, quality, and safety) of the care delivered to the population, and improve that performance as part of ongoing operations. This integration of quality improvement into regular operations requires centralized infrastructure and leadership.

In the next chapter, we will describe some of the systems that provider organizations use to perform these functions, but in this section we seek to fill out the vision of organized care so that the reader can recognize it as an attainable goal. Table 4.3 lists descriptions of how these aims might be fulfilled by an effective provider organization for four common types of patients—those with chronic disease (e.g., hypertension or diabetes), patients with complex conditions (e.g., combination of heart failure, cancer, and depression), the worried well, and the unworried well (i.e., people who are healthy and not actively engaged in improving their health). These snapshots are not a full description of any program but are intended to offer insight into what organized care might look like for different patients with different needs.

We want to highlight a few themes that characterize the snapshots in table 4.3. First, most of the provider investments that are needed to make these visions real are not directly supported by fee-for-service payments. Examples include communication with patients outside of

Table 4.3
Visions of care in organized delivery systems

	Patients with chronic diseases	Patients with complex conditions	Worried well	Unworried well
Safe	All key patient information is available to patients' clinicians	When patients are discharged from hospital, key information such as medications is conveyed to patients and their physicians	Patients have access to information on interactions between their prescribed medications and over-the-counter drugs	Patients are alerted immediately when one of their medications is recalled due to safety issues
Effective	Patients receive all treatments likely to reduce complications of their conditions (e.g., blood pressure control for diabetics)	Patients receive all treatments likely to reduce complications of their conditions after consideration of the impact of their other diseases	Patients and clinicians have shared understanding of preventive health goals	Patients receive reminders of need for key screening tests, and their compliance is monitored through tracking systems
Patient centered	Patients are actively engaged in management of their conditions	Patients' wishes regarding treatment plan including end-of-life care are sought and respected	Patients' concerns are heard and addressed	Patients are offered variety of options for working with providers
Timely	Patients returning for routine follow-up are seen without significant waits	Patients do not have unnecessary waiting for information, appointments, or treatments	Patients' questions are addressed by providers within twenty-four hours	Patients can access practice to ask questions and make requests by phone or email
Efficient	Patients are prescribed most cost-effective medications	Patients are followed by care coordination program to help reduce preventable hospital admissions	Patients receive education and follow-up rather than tests and medications unlikely to benefit them	Patients at risk for diabetes and other chronic conditions receive education on how to improve health prognosis

Table 4.3
(continued)

	Patients with chronic diseases	Patients with complex conditions	Worried well	Unworried well
Equitable	All patients are equally likely to receive treatments likely to be beneficial	All patients are offered treatments likely to be beneficial	Diverse provider organization offers welcoming setting for care	Culturally sensitive outreach programs are developed and implemented

reimbursed office visits and actual improvement in patients' control of their chronic diseases. Second, many of these snapshots imply easy and reliable interactions among various health care providers. For instance, for key information to be available to patients' various clinicians at any time and place, these clinicians must use information systems that communicate with each other. Finally, in organized care, the care is organized around the patient—not the physician. Note that the subject in most of the cells of table 4.3 is the patient. The measure of success in organization is whether the patients' needs are being met.

Concern over rising health care costs makes the fifth row on this table ("Efficiency") particularly important. With organized care, cost savings can result from the reduction of hospitalizations through the 24–7 availability of skilled professionals with access to patient's clinical information and more effective preventive care, especially among the patients with the highest risk for admission to severe or complex conditions. Efficiency can also result from improved physician decision making, such as can be encouraged through the use of computerized decision support that guides physicians to the most cost-effective tests and treatments. Organized systems can also make meaningful efforts to provide care in the most efficient settings—for example, outpatient versus inpatient, or community versus teaching hospital. In contrast, in a fragmented system, every entity tries to hold on to every patient.

The Patients' Perspectives

We now examine more deeply the requirements of effective provider organizations from the perspective of each of these four types of patients.

Patients with Chronic Disease

Diabetes, high blood pressure, high cholesterol, and many other chronic conditions are increasingly common as the U.S. population ages (and gains weight). To meet the needs of patients with these conditions, a provider organization must do more than offer physician visits at which the patient is examined and tests are obtained. From work within our own organization, we believe patients with chronic disease should have care that is:

• *Continuous*   Care should be available and useful throughout the year, not just during encounters with physicians. For example, hypertension is more likely to be controlled if patients can transmit frequent blood pressure readings from a home monitor into a database in which the readings can be monitored.

• *Collaborative*   Teams that include physicians and nonphysicians (e.g., nurses, nutritionists, and pharmacists) and patients themselves should work together to ensure that patients reach their clinical goals. For instance, patients with diabetes tend to have better rates of control of their glucose levels when they receive care not just from a doctor but also from a diabetes educator who may be allowed to adjust medication doses.

• *Informative*   For patients to play a major role in their own care, they must understand their conditions, their role, and how to track their progress. An insight that is still new for many physicians is that providing information is actually a form of care. This information should be available in a language and at an educational level that is understandable to these patients—a formidable standard that small physician practices rarely can meet.

• *Reliable*   Patients should have the opportunity to receive all of the care interventions that evidence suggests might be beneficial for them. If a patient is *not* receiving an important intervention, the reason should be documented in the patient's chart.

• *Safe*   Patient information should be available in a central EMR so that clinicians do not cause harm because they don't know what each other is doing.

• *Proactive*   Registries of populations of patients with chronic conditions should be maintained so that providers can reach out to patients who are falling short of their goals. For example, care teams should be able to identify the diabetics under their care who have poorly controlled blood pressure, glucose, and cholesterol levels. And then they should figure out how to work with those patients to do better.

Patients with Complex Medical Conditions

The sickest 5 percent of patients account for about 50 percent of health care spending, and the vast majority of these patients have more than one major medical issue. For example, they might have heart failure complicated by kidney disease and depression. Or they might have cancer complicated by diabetes and emphysema. And these medical problems may be worsened by poverty or chaotic circumstances in their home life.

A diabetes educator can only do so much for these patients, no two of whom are alike. They do not need *population*-based care (e.g., making sure all the diabetics get their eye exams). They need intensely *personalized* care that addresses their unique combination of issues—and they need plenty of it. Among the most successful interventions for these patients are nurses who are trained to be "care coordinators," who stay in frequent touch with patients in person and/or via telephone.

Care for these patients should be:

• *Continuous*   These patients are at high risk for being admitted to the hospital (or worse). On any given day, they may look sick enough that a physician who has never seen them before might want to admit them to the hospital. Thus, it is particularly important that these patients have a close relationship with a small group of clinicians—ideally a physician working with nonphysicians who are available 24–7.

• *Collaborative*   Teams of clinicians need to work with each other and the patient—and particularly in this population, the patient's family.

• *Informative*   The patients and their families need to be able to recognize early signs that a patient might be getting worse, so that problems can be addressed before they become too severe. They also need to have a realistic understanding of the patient's overall prognosis and treatment options.

• *Reliable*   The provider organization has to be ready when the patient reaches out for help—including at night and on weekends.

• *Safe*   Many of these patients get care from numerous physicians and institutions. The sharing of information among the involved clinicians is especially crucial. Patients should ideally try to keep their care within groups of physicians who all use the same EMR.

• *Proactive* The provider organization should not wait for these patients to call for help. Instead, someone should contact patients on a regular basis to check on how they are feeling, and monitor simple data like their blood pressure and weight.

The Worried Well
For these patients, a warm relationship with a primary care physician is just the starting point of what they want from their health care provider organization. Although they are not in any immediate danger, they want to know that they have access to help when they need it from someone who knows them. They pick up news from the Internet, and want to have a way to learn more and get their questions answered.

Information and ready access are exactly what many provider organizations are offering this subset. Patients in many organizations can do more than request appointments via the Internet; they can actually book their physician visits and key tests like mammograms. They can look into their EMRs and review their laboratory tests, and check for reminders of when they are due for preventive care interventions like Pap smears.

Many of these patients want control over their own care, and intelligent provider organizations are figuring out ways to give it to them.

The Unworried Well
Then there are the 20 percent of people who do not have any contact with the health care system in any given year. Many of them go years between physician visits, and some pride themselves on that. (They are not all male, but it sometimes seems that way.) The problem is that many of these unworried well are gaining weight, and have high blood pressure and other risk factors for heart attack and stroke. Some even know they have these problems, but do not seek care for financial, logistical, or psychological reasons.

An organized group of providers does not overlook these people, who might live a longer and healthier life if they get the right care. To reach out to them, organized providers need to know who is within their population—and that usually translates into which people are assigned to their primary care physicians. The provider organization needs a structure for tracking these populations, and calling in those who have not come in for their blood pressure checks, colorectal cancer screening, mammograms, and Pap smears.

The snapshots in table 4.3 and the descriptions of care that follow are not futuristic fantasies in which patients can magically find out everything they need to know through the Internet, physicians all communicate with each other, and nothing slips through the cracks. The fact is that many Americans already receive care that is this well coordinated, timely, and effective. The Americans who are most likely to get either part of or else this entire package are not necessarily those who have greater wealth or are more at ease with the Internet. The more critical factor is whether they receive their care from providers who are truly organized. Thus, a fundamental irony of U.S. health care today is that many people gravitate to the small, one or two doctor practice because they know the people there and staff remembers them. But when patients have to get care outside those small practices, it can feel like a trip to a foreign country without a passport.

Most Americans are not currently receiving care from well-organized providers, but some are. In the next chapter, we will describe some of the types of systems that are bringing organization to the care of more and more patients—and with it, better health.

5   What Kinds of Systems Improve Health Care?

Physicians, patients, and nurses sit in different spots in the health care system, but they all face one common impossible task. They are constantly bombarded by information, most of it mundane and reassuring. But some of those data are potentially ominous, and the consequences of missing warning signs or abnormal test results can be tragic.

The flood of information is overwhelming. Abnormal mammograms are occasionally overlooked. Medications are given even though patients have allergies to the drugs. Tests are repeated because the results from earlier examinations cannot be located. Patients leave the hospital or physicians' offices confused about what medications they should be taking and which doctors they should see next.

A basic problem that plagues health care is that these doctors, patients, and nurses are human. They try their best, but they make mistakes. Those mistakes frequently lead to wasted time and resources. Sometimes they endanger the health of patients.

Of course, doctors and nurses should be intelligent, hardworking, and well trained. But trying to fix our problems in health care by exhorting doctors and nurses to learn more and work harder only helps a little. To create real improvement, we need clinicians to interact with each other and their patients, and to do so using systems that improve coordination and reduce the risk of errors.

Some of these systems are electronic in nature—such as EMRs with decision support that helps physicians order the right drugs and tests. Some systems are humanware—such as teams of physicians and non-physicians that provide chronic care to patients with conditions like heart failure or complex medical conditions. For providers, these systems demand difficult cultural changes if they are to lead to meaningful improvements in care.

The first major change is an orientation toward error reduction. Physicians make hundreds of decisions per day based on their stored knowledge and clinical judgment. Because they cannot know everything they need to know, some of their decisions are not as efficient or safe as they could be. The use of information systems with decision support acknowledges that such errors occur, and that systems like EMRs might help physicians "get it right the first time." For example, if physicians have computerized decision support that guides them toward safe and cost-effective choices, there should be fewer calls from pharmacies to doctors' offices asking for the prescription to be changed.

A second cultural change is that these systems force everyone to speak the same language. The use of common systems mandates that clinicians interact with the world through the same "interfaces"; these systems simply won't work unless the clinicians use the same terminology as the rest of their colleagues—such as the same abbreviations for diagnoses like diabetes (AODM, which is short for "adult onset diabetes mellitus") and congestive heart failure (CHF). Common terminology is a basic requirement for communication, and communication is a basic requirement for collaboration.

The third and most fundamental change is the recognition of the importance of team care. Doctors cannot work alone in the care of complex patients with multiple conditions, and the truth is that they should not work alone in the care of other populations, including patients with chronic diseases, or people who are basically healthy and trying their best to remain that way. In effective provider organizations, physicians are members of teams that track and improve the care of populations (e.g., patients with diabetes), and also provide care to individual patients outside their physician office visits.

Many physicians complain that using EMRs and working with teams slows them down. In some instances, electronic records can actually reduce work for physicians by automating tasks like writing renewals of prescriptions. Yet in general, these systems do *not* reduce work for physicians. The truth is that electronic and human systems add *new types* of work to the physician's day, such as entering data into lists of medications and clinical problems, and answering emails from patients and colleagues.

Physicians are not happy about adding work to their already-difficult days, of course, but these new types of work can have considerable payoffs for patients. The work of entering information into the EMR leads to more reliable interactions among colleagues and with patients. These interactions (e.g., the sharing of knowledge of what medications a patient is taking) reduce the chances that doctors or patients will make mistakes, or that those mistakes will go undetected.

The use of electronic systems and teams including nonphysicians also creates new possibilities in efforts to make the patient a participant in their own care. For virtually all patients, the result of that collaboration should be a greater understanding of what they should be doing to improve their health. For the sickest and most complex patients, this collaboration can help them stay out of the hospital and possibly even live longer.

In this chapter, we will describe some key types of systems that have the potential to improve health care. We will first summarize the assessments made by two employer-led organizations (Bridges to Excellence and Leapfrog) of what systems matter most. We will then provide deeper descriptions of some of the key systems identified by these two groups. This information will set the stage for an examination in the next two chapters of the different types of delivery organizations that are using these systems to create order out of chaos.

What Systems Improve Care?

In 2001, the executives in charge of health care at General Electric (GE) were puzzling over the challenges of rising costs and disappointing quality, and decided they needed to try some new tactics. Up to that point, they had tried to act through health insurance plans. They demanded lower costs and better quality by using their "big stick" on the health plans: they threatened to move their business to other insurers. And they frequently did just that, earning as they did so a reputation among health insurance companies as the toughest of customers. Nevertheless, GE's health care costs continued to rise at about the same rate as everyone else's, and it couldn't detect much in the way of improved health for its employees.

GE's executives concluded that they needed to try a new approach, and decided to tackle these issues using the same methods that were so successful for the company's manufacturing and service industries in the 1990s. Robert S. Galvin, MD, and François de Brantes organized a "Six Sigma Design Team" of about a dozen people that included staff from GE Aircraft's plants in Cincinnati and Boston, along with health care providers and health plan representatives from the two regions.

The assignment: identify the key processes and systems that are most likely to lead to better care, so that GE and other employers could develop an incentive program to reward providers who used them.

To identify the processes and systems, the GE-led team applied the same Product Design for Six Sigma process that GE used for designing new aircraft engines and other products. In the GE world, this process was used so regularly that it was known by its initials—PDFSS. It is a disciplined, multistep process in which no individual's opinions can dominate. Moving relentlessly forward, this process develops group consensus on:

1. Who are the key "customers" for the product?

2. What matters most to those customers? (In Six Sigma lingo, what is "Critical to Quality"? For hard-core Six Sigma devotees, these key values are called "CTQs.")

3. Among the various values that are critical to quality, what are their relative "weights"? In other words, is cost more important than safety and reliability? Does timeliness count as much as safety?

4. Given the relative weights assigned to the various values, what processes and systems are most likely to create the most total value for the customer?

The design team (which included one of the authors, TL) considered patients to be the most important customers for health care. Physicians and other providers were considered "stakeholders" whose opinions mattered, but the design team was constantly reminded that the real goal was improving care for patients. The team adopted as critical to quality the six key aims for health care from the Institute of Medicine described in chapter 4: safety, effectiveness, patient centeredness, timeliness, efficiency, and equitableness. When relative weights were assigned to these six attributes, the aim of safety emerged as the most important, trailed closely by effectiveness and efficiency.

The design team concluded that physician practices could maximize the total value across these various attributes if they improved their ability to perform several crucial functions. Working with the NCQA, the Bridges to Excellence designers developed standards for physician practices' ability to [1]:

• Enable patients to communicate with and access the practice easily

• Use systems to track patients, along with their treatments and conditions

- Manage patients' care proactively over time
- Support patients' self-management of their health
- Use electronic prescribing tools
- Track and follow up lab and imaging tests
- Track and follow up referrals
- Measure performance, and work to improve it
- Update to interoperable electronic systems

The scoring system rewards physicians for implementing EMRs, and then using them fully (see next section). The program also rewards physicians for having humanware systems in place to keep track of their highest-risk patient populations, and providing ready access to health care information and the practice itself for all patients, regardless of their condition. The actual system used to score practices on whether or not they have implemented these systems can be accessed through the NCQA's Web site (<http://www.ncqa.org>).

Bridges to Excellence is oriented toward improving the care delivered in physician offices; its hospital-oriented counterpart is another organization started by employers, Leapfrog (<http://www.leapfrog-group.org/home>). Leapfrog reports data on hospitals via its Web site on several characteristics that it believes contribute to better quality and efficiency, including:

Computerized Physician Order Entry (CPOE) That is, does the hospital require its staff to use computers to order medications, tests, and procedures?

Intensive Care Unit (ICU) Staffing That is, does the hospital have an ICU that is staffed by doctors and other caregivers who have special training in critical care (also known as intensivists)?

High-Risk Treatments That is, does the hospital perform a reasonable volume of operations like coronary artery bypass graft surgery and bariatric surgery, and does it have good outcomes?

Leapfrog Safe Practices Score That is, how does the hospital compare with others on the use of twenty-seven procedures that can be expected to reduce preventable medical mistakes?

The common themes of Bridges to Excellence and Leapfrog are the emphases on the use of information systems and effective interactions among teams of clinicians to provide coordinated, efficient, and safe care. Although some providers have resisted the notion that employers should be defining excellence for doctors and hospitals, both programs are widely respected for the thought behind their measures and their overall impact. Based on these assessments from Bridges to Excellence and Leapfrog, we now go deeper in exploring some of the key systems most likely to bring organization and improvement to health care.

EMRs

EMRs are not in themselves a miracle cure for health care's problems. Indeed, skeptics like to point out that definitive evidence that EMRs improve quality or efficiency is scant [2]. Yet the design team of Bridges to Excellence concluded that major improvement in health care simply cannot occur without physicians making a transition from paper medical records to computerized EMRs—and we agree.

From the perspective of patients, the only obvious change when their physicians "go electronic" may be that the doctors spend less time flipping through paper charts in search of information—and more time looking at a computer screen. For clinicians, however, EMRs have several well-defined critical functions (table 5.1) [3].

A basic EMR is able to collect and store information about patients, and enables clinicians to retrieve these data when needed. If physicians order tests and medications through their EMR, it should be able to guide them to the safest and most reliable choices. And the EMR should help physicians and their colleagues do a better job of keeping track of patients' needs than is possible for an individual physician using a paper chart.

An extensive survey conducted in late 2007 and early 2008 found that only 4 percent of U.S. physicians had fully functional EMRs, and

Table 5.1
Functionalities of an electronic health record system

Core functionalities*	Other functionalities
1. Health information and data	1. Electronic communication and connectivity
2. Results management	2. Patient support
3. Order entry and support	3. Administrative support
4. Decision support	4. Reporting and population health management

Note: *These categories were determined by an advisory panel to the federal government's Health Information Technology Adoption Initiative to be the core functionalities of an electronic health record. (Table reproduced with permission from [3].)

another 13 percent had more basic systems [4]. This survey found that primary care physicians and those practicing in large groups or medical centers were more likely to use EMRs. Financial barriers were the biggest obstacle to EMRs, and older physicians were slightly less likely to be EMR users.

Although EMR users were in the minority among U.S. physicians, they were for the most part pleased with the impact of EMRs on their care—and they felt that more advanced systems had a greater impact. Figure 5.1 shows that physicians who had fully functional electronic records systems were more likely to report positive effects from their EMR on the quality of clinical decisions (82 percent), communication with other providers (92 percent) and patients (72 percent), prescription refills (95 percent), timely access to medical records (97 percent), and avoidance of medication errors (86 percent). These physicians were also more likely to report that their EMR helped them comply with preventive and chronic care guidelines. Physicians with basic

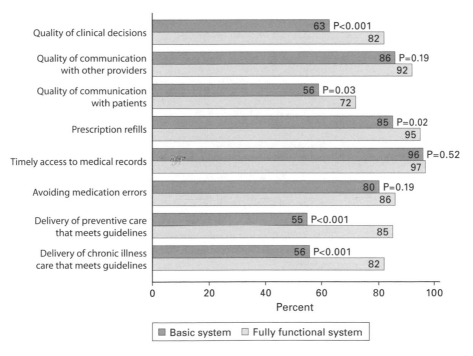

Figure 5.1
Rates of positive survey responses on the effect of adoption of electronic health records systems. (Reproduced with permission from the *New England Journal of Medicine*)

systems reported benefits as well, but the impact was generally smaller.

How exactly do EMRs yield these benefits? Let's list some of the major types of problems described in the first chapters of this book, and consider the potential of EMRs to address them (table 5.2).

To illustrate practical examples of how EMRs can help address these problems, we provide some screen shots from the EMR developed by our organization, Partners HealthCare System. (Because of privacy concerns, these screen shots come from the record of an imaginary "test" forty-three-year-old female, not a real patient.) Figure 5.2 shows

Table 5.2
Ten problems, and how EMRs potentially address them

Problems	How EMRs potentially address them
1. Too much to do	EMRs can keep track of key tests and treatments that patients should receive, and remind physicians and other team members to act
2. Too much patient information to track	EMRs can organize test results and other data, and alert clinicians if there are worrisome findings
2. Too much to know	EMRs can provide clinicians instant access to information from textbooks and journals
4. Too little time	EMRs can make it easier for physicians to work with nurses and other clinical personnel, who can assume work that does not require a doctor and provide care to patients outside the office visit
5. Too many physicians involved	EMRs make it easier for numerous physicians (who may be at multiple institutions) to share information and coordinate their efforts on behalf of complex patients
6. Rising healthcare costs	Physicians who prescribe medications and order tests through EMRs can receive decision support that guides them to the most cost-effective choices
7. Epidemic of safety problems	Decision support can prevent physicians from making errors, such as prescribing a medication that might be dangerous for a patient
8. The 24-7-365 culture	EMRs make information available to physicians and other members of the care team (potentially including the patient) at any time, and from any place
9. Patients are confused, and have trouble getting their questions answered	An increasing number of EMRs provide access to patients, so they can verify their medication lists; request referrals, appointments, and prescriptions; and even check their laboratory test results
10. The unworried well	EMRs can remind clinicians to contact people who do *not* come in for preventive care, but should

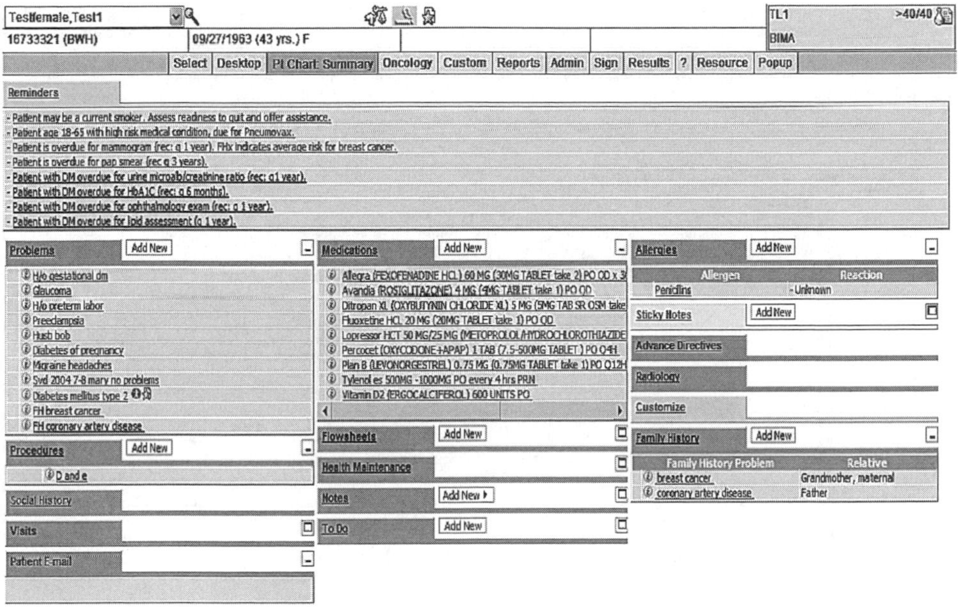

Figure 5.2
Summary screen for imaginary patient from EMR of Partners HealthCare System.

the summary screen that appears when the patient's record is opened. The small icons at the top remind the physician of key information. The stork figure provides direct access to a summary of her obstetric history. The box with a smoking cigarette indicates that the patient is an active smoker. The star on the rectangle offers direct access to a "smart form" that makes it easier for physicians to collect data and provide care for patients with diabetes.

The reminder section on the upper-left portion of the screen prompts physicians to supply a variety of preventive interventions likely to benefit a patient with the patient's medical problems. In the middle of the screen is a list of the patient's medications. Note the circles with an italicized "i." If users of the EMR click on these buttons, they are connected to a variety of information relevant to that drug or medical problem.

For example, if one were to click on the circle next to the medication "Avandia," the screen shown in figure 5.3 appears. Safety concerns regarding this medication for diabetes emerged in 2007, and clinicians were able to access the latest statements from the FDA through this EMR. Note on the left side of this screen the button with the

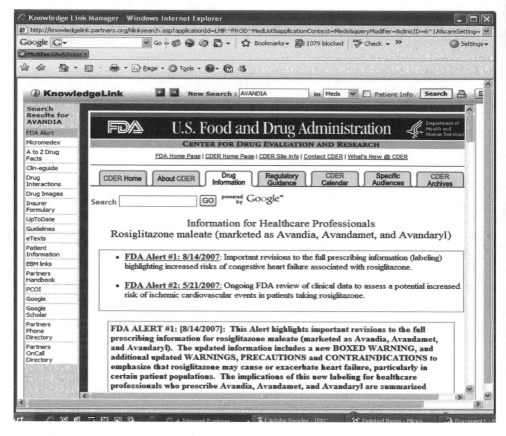

Figure 5.3
Example of information on Avandia accessible through Partners HealthCare System's
EMR.

title "Drug Images." Clicking on this box would take the viewer to
photos of the pill in question—a useful tool when physicians and
patients are trying to sort out exactly what medications the patient is
actually taking at home.

Figure 5.4 below shows what appears when a physician uses this
EMR to order Nexium, a medication that reduces acid secretion in
the stomach. Nexium is a fine drug, but there are numerous less
expensive alternatives available, including over-the-counter preparations that cost most patients less than they would have to pay when
filling a Nexium prescription. On-screen, the red dots on the left side
of the screen indicate that Nexium is a drug that should be used only

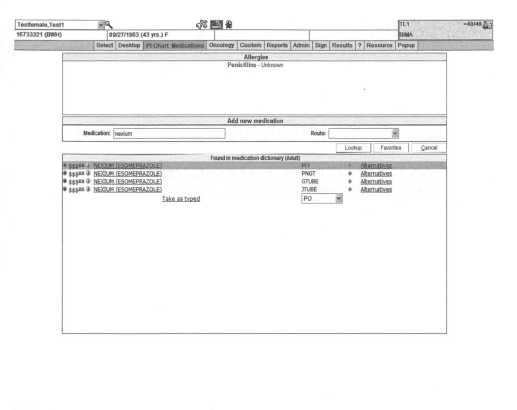

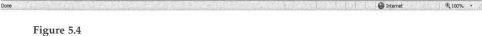

Figure 5.4
Screen shot that appears when Partners physicians order Nexium.

after drugs with green or yellow dots have been considered. The three dollar signs mean that the cost to the patient will be high. The "pa" means that for this patient's insurance plan, Nexium cannot be prescribed unless the physician completes a "Prior Authorization" form and gets approval from the insurer. The form can be printed out if the physician clicks on the letters "pa." But usually physicians will find it easier to click on the word "Alternatives" on the right side of the screen, taking them to the screen shot shown in figure 5.5. On-screen, green dots appear next to the most cost-effective options, which work well for the vast majority of patients—for example, omeprazole, the generic version of the brand-name drug Prilosec. Thus, this EMR makes it easier for physicians to know when they are prescribing a medication that is not covered by the patient's insurer

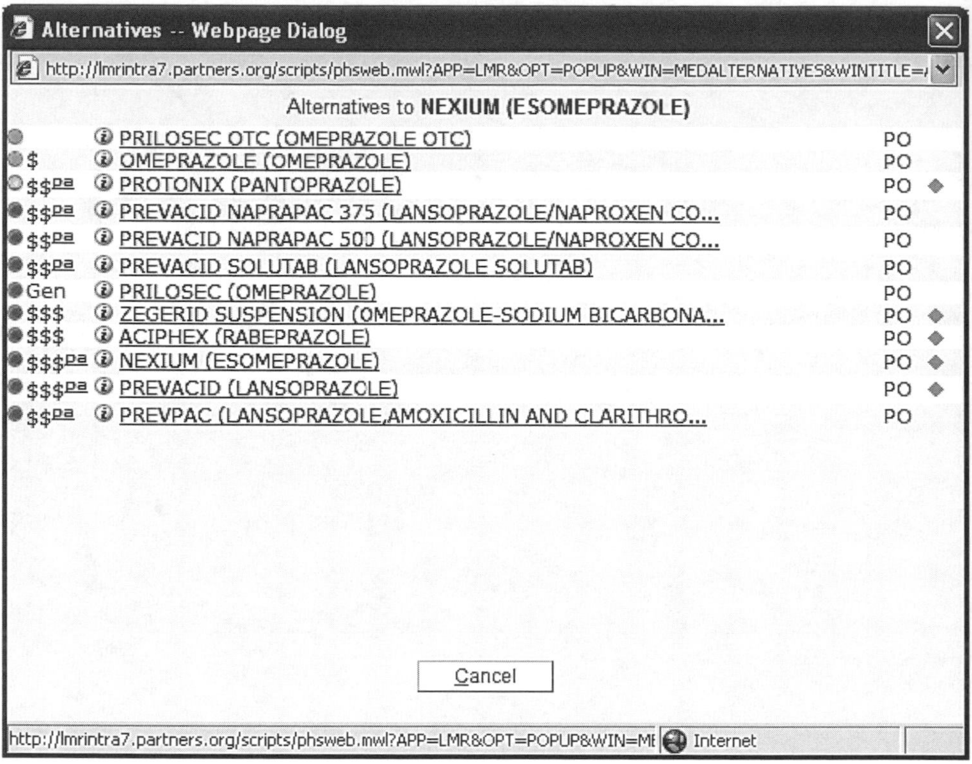

Alternatives -- Webpage Dialog [×]

http://lmrintra7.partners.org/scripts/phsweb.mwl?APP=LMR&OPT=POPUP&WIN=MEDALTERNATIVES&WINTITLE=/ ⌄

Alternatives to **NEXIUM (ESOMEPRAZOLE)**

●	ⓘ PRILOSEC OTC (OMEPRAZOLE OTC)	PO	
●$	ⓘ OMEPRAZOLE (OMEPRAZOLE)	PO	
○$$ᵖᵃ	ⓘ PROTONIX (PANTOPRAZOLE)	PO	◆
●$$ᵖᵃ	ⓘ PREVACID NAPRAPAC 375 (LANSOPRAZOLE/NAPROXEN CO...	PO	
●$$ᵖᵃ	ⓘ PREVACID NAPRAPAC 500 (LANSOPRAZOLE/NAPROXEN CO...	PO	
●$$ᵖᵃ	ⓘ PREVACID SOLUTAB (LANSOPRAZOLE SOLUTAB)	PO	
●Gen	ⓘ PRILOSEC (OMEPRAZOLE)	PO	
●$$$	ⓘ ZEGERID SUSPENSION (OMEPRAZOLE-SODIUM BICARBONA...	PO	◆
●$$$	ⓘ ACIPHEX (RABEPRAZOLE)	PO	◆
●$$$ᵖᵃ	ⓘ NEXIUM (ESOMEPRAZOLE)	PO	◆
●$$$ᵖᵃ	ⓘ PREVACID (LANSOPRAZOLE)	PO	◆
●$$ᵖᵃ	ⓘ PREVPAC (LANSOPRAZOLE,AMOXICILLIN AND CLARITHRO...	PO	

[Cancel]

http://lmrintra7.partners.org/scripts/phsweb.mwl?APP=LMR&OPT=POPUP&WIN=ME 🌐 Internet

Figure 5.5
Alternatives to Nexium.

or will be costly for the patient, and then to switch to a lower-cost, comparable agent.

Figure 5.6 provides an example of how this EMR helps physicians and their team members follow populations of patients with chronic diseases during and in between office visits. This screen shot comes from the actual population of diabetics followed by one of the authors (TL)—thus, the names, dates of birth, and medical record numbers of the patients are obscured. In the actual EMR, the physician can click on the patients' names and go directly into their records.

The graph at the top shows how many patients in his panel have varying degrees of control of their blood sugar levels. Levels of this test, hemoglobin A1c, are under seven in patients with good control of their diabetes. On the other hand, levels of nine or higher indicate poor control, which is associated with higher rates of complications from

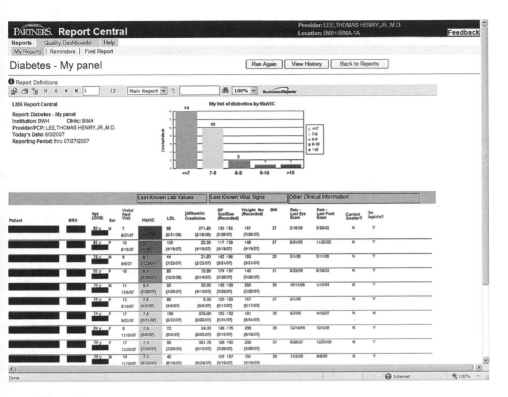

Figure 5.6
Screen shot of data summary on patients with diabetes under care of one physician.

diabetes. The table below depicts other key clinical information on the patients with poorly controlled diabetes, including their next scheduled office visit. The blank under "Next Visit" for the fourth patient means no visit for that patient is scheduled—which led this physician to contact this patient to ask her to come in for an appointment.

As these examples show, the information and tools within EMRs have the *potential* to improve the decisions made by individual physicians, and help them work more effectively with patients and other clinicians to care for patients with chronic diseases. But how great is this potential, and is it being realized? And because of the crisis in health care costs, what is the potential of EMRs to reduce health care spending?

There have been several studies of the potential impact of EMRs and their component functions (e.g., electronic prescribing), and the results have been mixed. Two widely cited studies estimated that national savings to the health care sector of $80 billion per year (in 2005 dollars) might be achievable with the optimal use of health information technology including EMRs [5–8]. These analyses, however, emphasized that these were *potential* savings that were based on optimistic interpretations of what was possible in ideal circumstances.

A CBO study from 2008 titled "Evidence on the Costs and Benefits of Health Information Technology" had a more sobering perspective, but saw a close connection between the impact of EMRs and provider organization. The CBO paper concluded that on its own, the adoption of information technologies generally does not produce significant cost savings. Nevertheless, the CBO paper concluded that health information technology including EMRs appear "to make it easier to reduce health spending if other steps in the broader health care system are also taken to alter incentives to promote savings" [2].

This CBO paper went on to note that the greatest impact of health information technology has been in "relatively integrated" provider systems, and cited Kaiser Permanente, Intermountain Health Care, Geisinger Health System, and Partners HealthCare as examples. (These and other systems are described in chapters 6 and 7.) At Kaiser Permanente, for instance, the introduction of EMRs has been associated with a 9 percent drop in office visits by its membership [9]. Kaiser Permanente physicians are not rewarded financially for generating more office visits, so EMR use in ways that help patients stay healthy without needing face-to-face contact with their physicians is in everyone's interest. On the other hand, the CBO report noted that "for providers and hospitals that are not part of integrated systems, however, the benefits of health IT are not as easy to capture, and perhaps not coincidentally, those physicians and facilities have adopted [EMRs] at a much slower rate" [2].

A reasonable perspective on EMRs is that they are necessary but not sufficient for high quality and improved efficiency—that is, EMRs are likely to be essential for major advances in addressing our various challenges, but the EMRs will have to improve, and clinicians will have to become sophisticated in their use. That sophistication does not come all at once.

Quality improvement leaders at Kaiser and other provider organizations now use a phased approach in their effort to improve care through EMR use. In the first phase, the EMR serves as a charting documentation tool that improves care in large part because it is legible and also reliably available to multiple physicians participating in a patient's care. In the second phase, the EMR begins to improve compliance with practice guidelines through the use of automated reminders. In the latter phases, more advanced functions provide new benefits, including electronic prescribing, access to the EMR from anywhere, and the integration of quality improvement programs into physicians' documentation tools. In a more recent phase that is being explored in many organizations, patients can get access to parts of the EMR, such as lab tests and medication lists, and the EMR can improve the collaboration between doctors and patients.

The sequence in which these phases are explored varies from organization to organization, and some physicians do not progress much beyond phases one or two. But the potential of EMRs to change the nature of health care is not lost on those who work with them.

What are the barriers that prevent most U.S. physicians from adopting EMRs? As reported in the 2007–2008 survey [4], the first and foremost problem is the cost, which ranges from $15,000 to $50,000 per physician. These costs are particularly high for physicians in solo or small group practices because the expenses cannot be spread over multiple doctors. The software licenses are relatively minor expenses compared to the costs of hardware, the connections to a local network and the Internet, and the training of staff. EMRs can lead to some savings, such as lower personnel costs related to the handling of paper medical records [2]. But small practices may not be able to realize these savings, because if they only have a few employees, they may not be able to eliminate any positions as a result of implementing EMRs.

A second problem is that the use of EMRs tends to slow physicians down. Doctors who have been jotting quick notes on paper as they talked to patients or scrawling prescriptions on pads for years are frustrated by the delays associated with stepping up to a computer terminal, logging on, and typing in notes and prescriptions. In addition, through their various reminders, EMRs prompt physicians to do a more complete job—which of course takes more time.

From a big picture perspective, EMRs help physicians deliver better care and also communicate what they are doing to their colleagues, and they even save doctors time by reducing phone calls from other doctors and pharmacies. Yet physicians are much more aware of the additional time required for tasks that used to take a few seconds, and many complain that the adoption of EMRs lengthens their day and raises their costs, without necessarily increasing their revenues.

Although we personally know many physicians who complain about EMRs, we do not know of any examples of physicians who have implemented an EMR and then gone back to paper charts. EMRs are expensive and can take more time, but they are so clearly supportive of better patient care that most physicians agree they cannot imagine reverting to paper.

CPOE

Now let's turn from physicians' offices to hospitals, where the risks of inadvertent injury to patients are the highest because so many interventions are being performed on the frailest of the frail. The hospital equivalent of electronic prescribing is CPOE, computerized ordering systems with decision support.

CPOE is in place in only a small percentage of U.S. hospitals, and the expense and disruption of implementing it are tremendous burdens for an industry that is already plagued by many problems. Investing millions of dollars does not guarantee that CPOE implementation will go smoothly—and in one spectacular 2003 failure, Cedars Sinai Hospital in Los Angeles stopped its CPOE implementation and went back to pen-and-paper systems for physician orders. But gradually, hospital by hospital, CPOE is spreading, and hospitals that do *not* have CPOE will likely be the exception rather than the rule sometime in the next decade.

The major reason for CPOE's steady spread is the fear of medication errors—patients receiving the wrong drug or getting a drug in the wrong dose. Sometimes physicians order a drug to which the patient is allergic or one that has a dangerous interaction with another medication. At other times, the physician's handwriting is illegible, or the doctor's memory of the correct amount or frequency of the medication may be faulty.

Hospitals with CPOE use electronic prescribing systems that intercept errors—ideally at the moment that the physician enters them into the computer. Some hospitals accommodate older physicians who are not comfortable with computers or facile with typing, and have nonphysicians transcribe doctors' handwritten orders. At some point, though, the logic programmed into the CPOE system can screen the orders to see if they make sense and are likely to be safe for the patient.

Research suggests that CPOE has the potential to reduce medication errors by half or more [10], but much of that research comes from one hospital (Brigham and Women's Hospital, which is part of the authors' health care delivery system). And some data have shown that CPOE systems have the ability to *cause* errors if used improperly [11]. Nevertheless, most hospitals want to implement CPOE because serious medication errors are horrifying experiences for their staff, and have major potential adverse public relations and malpractice consequences. Just as improvement of the office practice of medicine is difficult to imagine in the absence of EMRs, CPOE is seen as an essential step toward developing safer hospitals.

CPOE has the potential to improve more than safety. The decision support within CPOE systems can guide physicians toward more efficient medication and test choices. Hospitals can also improve the reliability with which they provide interventions for specific patient populations if they identify those patients via the initial set of orders entered into the CPOE system.

For example, if the physician who is writing the initial set of orders for the patient has to choose among coded admitting diagnoses, the hospital staff can immediately identify patients with heart failure, heart attacks, or pneumonia. They can also identify patients who are cigarette smokers. By tracking these populations of patients from the moment they arrive, the hospital can ensure that they receive all the interventions likely to be beneficial to them during the hospitalization and afterward (e.g., beta-blockers for patients who have had heart attacks, smoking cessation counseling for cigarette smokers, and so on).

CPOE can be used to reduce confusion about what medications the patient should be taking after they have been discharged from the hospital as well. At our hospitals, we are "hardwiring" our order entry systems so that it is impossible to discharge patients without the physician reviewing the lists of medications that the patient was taking before and during the hospital admission—and giving a single clear list of what the patient should be taking, and ensuring that physicians who provide outpatient care to the patient know why certain medications may have been stopped.

In table 5.3, we describe ten common inpatient problems and how CPOE can be used to address them.

Despite these potential benefits, CPOE implementation is proceeding slowly and painfully. The cost is several million dollars at most institutions, and the disruption to the routines of busy physicians is an even more formidable challenge. CPOE, however, is seen by

Table 5.3
Ten common inpatient problems, and how CPOE systems address them

Problem	How CPOE systems address them
1. Patient allergic to prescribed medication	If allergies are known and entered into information system, CPOE can alert prescribing physician
2. Drug interacts with another medication	If all medications are ordered through CPOE, software can detect potentially dangerous interactions
3. Wrong drug given because doctor's handwriting is illegible	CPOE systems require typed entry of medications
4. Doctor enters dose ten times too high	CPOE systems can alert physicians ordering medication outside of usual dosage range
5. Dosage should be adjusted for certain patients	Some CPOE systems recommend dose adjustments for patients with characteristics that affect the potency of specific drugs; examples of such characteristics include advanced age and kidney disease
6. Too much to do	"Templates" of orders approved by local experts can be used to ensure that patients with specific diagnoses receive key interventions
7. Too much to know	Physicians can access information resources such as textbooks and medical journals as they enter orders
8. Rising health care costs	CPOE systems can guide physicians to more cost-effective choices of drugs and tests
9. Patients do not receive all recommended care	CPOE systems can be used to identify populations of patients such as cigarette smokers and those with heart disease, and ensure they receive recommended interventions during and after discharge
10. Patients confused about postdischarge care	CPOE systems can be used to ensure that medication regimens and other key postdischarge plans are carefully thought through and communicated to patient

Leapfrog and others as a key component of a better health care system, and information on whether or not hospitals have CPOE is now readily available in most markets. With such pressures, an increasing number of hospitals are implementing CPOE, despite the cultural challenges and cost.

Safe Electronic Medication Administration Systems

About half of the medication errors in hospitals occur at the time that physicians write the orders; these should be greatly reduced through the spread of CPOE systems. But a comparable proportion of medication errors occur *after* the physician has written a correct order. A tragic example of such errors cost the lives of three infants who were given fatal overdoses of the blood-thinning medication heparin at an Indianapolis hospital in 2006.

As reported on September 24, 2006, by the *Indianapolis Star*, the first misstep was made by a pharmacy technician who mistakenly supplied the medication cabinet of the neonatal intensive care unit (NICU) with heparin in vials usually used for adults. Because of their greater body size, adults need higher doses of heparin to prevent blood clots, so the medication vials for adults contain much more concentrated preparations of the drug than the vials normally used for the tiny infants in the NICU. It was an innocent error by a technician with twenty-five years of experience.

The heparin vials for adults and infants looked different, but not that different. The adult vials were dark blue; the NICU vials were light blue. The adult vials said, "Heparin"; the NICU vials said, "Hep-Lock." The vials were the same size. Five different NICU nurses mistakenly gave six different infant patients heparin from the adult vials. Once they recognized the error, they gave a drug that reverses the effects of heparin, but were only able to save three of the six infants.

The Indianapolis hospital, Methodist Hospital, did not fire any of the personnel involved. Instead, the hospital accepted the blame for the errors, saying that it did not have sufficient safeguards in place. It began to require that its pharmacy double check all drugs leaving its stockrooms, and that two nurses check the doses of medications given to infants. And the hospital accelerated its implementation of a new system to scan bar codes on medications and patient identification bracelets, to be sure that the right patient was getting the right drug in the right dose at the right time.

Although these safe medication administration systems have not attracted as much public attention as CPOE, they are the next frontier for hospitals on the leading edge of promoting patient safety. These systems attracted even more attention in 2007, when twin newborns of the actor Dennis Quaid and his wife suffered heparin overdoses because of a similar type of mistake. As will be described in the next chapter, the Veterans Health Administration began implementing safe medication administration systems after a nurse observed that car rental agencies did more with bar codes to track their cars than her hospital did with medications. A modest number of hospitals around the country are now going down the same road—in some cases, tragically, after catastrophic errors such as occurred in Indianapolis.

The major components of these systems include:

1. The bar coding of medications, down to individual pills and intravenous bag solutions

2. The bar coding of identification bracelets of patients

3. The bar coding on the identification badges of hospital personnel

4. A wireless system that allows nurses at the bedside to scan the medication and patient's identification bracelet to ensure that the correct patient is receiving the right drug in the dose ordered (ideally via the hospital's CPOE system)

Implementing these systems is a major expense for hospitals. Their pharmacies must develop processes for the bar coding of single doses of medications or work with an outside contractor to perform this function (at costs of about eleven to twenty cents per pill). The hospital has to install a wireless network, and buy laptop computers and scanners to be placed on stands that can be steered to the patients' bedsides. The nurses have to take the time to scan the medication and identification bracelet of the patient, and get the go-ahead signal from the computer system before giving the patient the drug.

Compared to the older, simpler way of giving patients a medication in a hospital—that is, a nurse would bring a patient a small white cup with his or her pills—all this bar coding and scanning at the bedside might seem to be a lot of fuss to prevent a few errors. But no one is questioning whether these systems are worth implementing in Indianapolis. Most nurses who use these systems quickly learn how many errors are prevented. They comment that making a medication error is perhaps their greatest single fear, and nurses have turned into the biggest advocates for these systems at many hospitals.

Why isn't every hospital moving to adopt such safe medication administration systems? One major reason is that until recently, there has been no direct financial justification for the huge required investments. Some pay-for-performance contracts are beginning to reward hospitals for adopting these systems, though, and the public reporting of serious medication errors is gaining support in many regions— further increasing the pressure on hospitals to take on this challenging task.

Care Coordination for Patients with Chronic Diseases

Physicians are excellent at reacting. A patient shows up at an office or emergency department in pain, and doctors go into action, figure out what is causing the symptoms, and start treatments to relieve them. Patients have a question, and physicians give an answer. The phone rings or the beeper goes off, and physicians respond.

Physicians do so much reacting, there isn't much time or energy left for being proactive—that is, dealing with anything other than the problem screaming for attention. That means most doctors do not routinely look over the list of their patients with diabetes to see who has not had their eye examinations, teach overweight patients about diets that might reduce the chances of a heart attack or stroke in two or three decades, or contact patients who have not shown up for their follow-up office visits. Many physicians provide this kind of care for some of their patients, but few practices are set up to do so for *all* of their patients who stand to benefit from it.

Yet this sort of proactive care aimed at preventing problems in the future is just what patients with chronic diseases and complex medical conditions need if they are to reduce their risk of hospitalizations and premature death. Since these patients account for most of the health care costs in the United States, systems to care for patients in between their visits to physicians are a critical part of organized health care. These systems focus on improving the outlook of *populations* of high-risk patients by caring for them throughout the year, rather than solely concentrating on addressing the symptoms of the *individual* sitting in front of the doctor.

Two basic approaches are gaining increasingly common use: the chronic care model, and disease management. These approaches overlap, but there are sufficient differences in their target populations and tactics that they warrant separate descriptions.

Chronic Care Model   Many patients with medical conditions like diabetes, heart failure, high blood pressure, and asthma feel fine on any given day. When their chronic diseases cause crises, like strokes, heart attacks, or severe shortness of breath, these patients go to the doctor or emergency department, and physicians then do what they can to help. But truly excellent care for these patients includes helping them control their medical conditions so that such crises are prevented or at least delayed.

The tension between excellent chronic care and the focus of the physicians on acute illnesses has been called "the Tyranny of the Urgent" [12]. When doctors are preoccupied with acute illnesses, visits are brief, and patients are not adequately taught to care for themselves. Nonphysician personnel are generally not available to help the physician meet patients' longer-term needs. As one group of authors put it, "Too often, caring for chronic illness features an uninformed passive patient interacting with an unprepared practice team, resulting in frustrating, inadequate encounters" [12].

The most widely used model for helping patients with chronic conditions was described by Edward H. Wagner, MD, who helps design systems to care for such patients at the Group Health Cooperative of Puget Sound, an HMO in Seattle. Wagner's model requires effective interaction among six essential elements of the health care system and community:

1. *Community resources and policies*   To improve chronic care, provider organizations should have linkages to community resources such as senior centers, exercise programs, and self-help groups.

2. *Health care systems*   Health insurers need to provide financial rewards for improving chronic care, and health care providers need to respond.

3. *Self-management support*   Patients need to assume the role of principal caregivers. They need to understand their conditions, and monitor their success in controlling their weight, blood pressure, blood sugar, and other factors that lead to risk for complications. To help patients acquire these skills, the health care system needs to offer education and tools (e.g., devices for monitoring blood pressure) to patients and their families.

4. *Delivery system design*   The medical practice has to be redesigned to accommodate functions besides putting sick patients in front of their doctors. Important components of organized care systems include nonphysician personnel trained in supporting patient self-management and systems to track populations of patients with chronic diseases.

5. *Decision support*   Physicians, other clinicians, and patients need reminders of when patients need eye exams, blood tests, and other interventions. These reminders can be conveyed through computerized information systems or paper-based ones.

6. *Clinical information systems* Paper systems can remind clinicians to perform certain functions when the patient's chart is being reviewed during an office visit, but computerized information systems are needed to track populations and prompt care when a patient is not there. These computerized systems allow for the development of registries—databases of all patients with a specific condition, with data on who needs which intervention.

The chronic care model has been implemented in part or whole within numerous well-structured delivery organizations, and there is strong evidence that such organizations improve the health of patients with chronic conditions [13]. The evidence on whether the chronic care model can save costs is less clear. There are reasonably convincing studies showing that congestive heart failure programs can lower costs while improving patients' quality of life and survival, and some studies have found lower costs with such care for patients with asthma and diabetes. The cost savings are usually achieved by reducing rates of emergency department visits and hospitalizations.

But for all these conditions, some studies have *failed* to find cost savings sufficiently large to offset the costs of the programs themselves. In addition, the cost savings are not always enjoyed by the organizations paying for the programs that improve these patients' care. Under the traditional fee-for-service payment system, for example, a provider organization that invests in programs that prevent physician visits and hospitalizations actually reduces its revenue.

Disease Management The phrase disease management is often applied to chronic care improvement efforts like those described in the preceding section, but this term is used more specifically to describe programs that involve repeated direct contact with a subset of patients with the highest risk for hospitalizations and complications. Chronic care improvement programs might cover the 20 to 25 percent of patients in a physicians' practice with chronic medical conditions. But disease management programs tend to focus on the 3 to 5 percent of patients who account for 45 to 50 percent of health care costs.

Disease management programs that involve direct contact with high-risk patients frequently rely on call centers with trained nurses who contact patients on a regular basis. Because the costs of such centers are high, these programs are usually run by for-profit companies that have contracts with health insurance plans. These companies analyze administrative data to identify patients who might be at high risk for hospitalization, and then nurses interview the patients to determine whether regular telephonic follow-up might be able to reduce that risk. If the patient agrees, the nurse will call the patient periodically and send the patient information (e.g., pamphlets or DVDs) about their medical condition.

These disease management nurses sometimes identify patients whose conditions are worsening, and encourage them to see their physicians before an emergency department visit or hospitalization is needed. Their other key function is the education of patients and their families on how to improve their self-management skills. Some provide Internet-based tools for tracking their conditions.

Do disease management programs save money? Data on their effectiveness as a cost-saving strategy are mixed. For example, a RAND study released in December 2007 analyzed the results of 317 different studies of disease management, and found consistent evidence that these programs can improve the quality of care, and in the case of patients with congestive heart failure, can reduce hospital admission rates [14]. But they actually found that patients with depression who were enrolled in disease management programs were *more* likely to use outpatient care and prescription drugs, thereby increasing costs. There is also uncertainty about whether these programs improve health outcomes for patients over the long term.

Nevertheless, insurance plans and large employers think that disease management is a good enough bet that they have signed large contracts with disease management companies (the total value of these contracts equaled about $1.2 billion in 2005). There is a strong sense among those who work in this field that years of work will be needed before conclusions can be drawn about the impact of disease management. These programs are likely to evolve and become increasingly integrated with physicians through their EMRs. And they are likely to develop more effective ways of staying in touch with patients, such as through their cell phones, or via Internet connections to their computers and even their bathroom scales.

An oft-used joke is, "Disease management is the future of medicine. . . . And it always will be." On the one hand, that joke demonstrates that disease management has yet to deliver on its promise. On the other hand, it conveys the message that no one should give up on disease management any time soon.

While the chronic care model was designed to improve the care offered by physicians and other providers, disease management companies interact directly with patients. Thus, disease management is usually carved out from the regular health care delivery system. Small physician practices cannot afford call centers and the other tools of disease management programs.

As summarized in a commentary by Lawrence Casalino [15],

Disease management companies are strong where most medical groups are weak: they have sophisticated information technology systems, arrays of data collected from multiple sources, predictive modeling software to identify chronically ill patients, well-developed processes for conducting disease management, and specially trained managers and staff whose focus is the companies' core competence—disease management. The disease management industry appears to have economies of scale far beyond the size of all but the largest physician groups—once modeling software, a biometric device, or a Web-based system for communicating with patients has been developed, it costs little to add thousands more patients.

Physician groups lack these advantages, but do have direct personal knowledge of their patients—knowledge they could potentially use in conjunction with whatever information technology systems and data they possess to help construct registries. Physicians can conduct in-person group visits, and more generally, can use their relationship with patients to promote cooperation with self-management and case management processes.

Is there a way to integrate the strengths of the chronic care model with those of disease management? Yes, but that requires physicians and other providers to be part of effective organizations. In the next chapter, we describe some providers who are demonstrating the potential of well-organized care.

6 Tightly Structured Health Care Delivery Organizations

Organized health care is not an abstract concept, a fantasy, or an unattainable ideal. In fact, millions of Americans already benefit from health care organizations that use information systems and teams of clinicians to provide safe, reliable, and efficient care. Many of the patients who use these organizations are unaware of the advantages that their systems offer—until those patients leave, and rediscover what health care is like when physicians do not share the same medical records, when letters and lab tests get lost on a regular basis, and when there are no processes that address their needs in between doctor visits. Once you have had well-organized health care, the acceptance of anything less is difficult.

Some of the best-organized health care providers in the United States have familiar names, but many do not. Even when the names are well-known, they are not necessarily the most prestigious in U.S. medicine. The Veterans Health Administration (VHA, or as it is also known, VA), for example, was ridiculed in movies in the post-Vietnam era because the care it provided was considered so poor; today, the VHA leads the country on many measures of quality of care. In contrast, many Americans have never heard of Geisinger Health System, the northeast Pennsylvania delivery organization with an innovative approach to coronary artery bypass graft (CABG) surgery that was featured in a front-page story in the *New York Times* in May 2007.

In this chapter, we will describe four tightly structured delivery organizations that are defining organized care and its benefits for the country. We call these organizations "tight" because they own their hospitals and other facilities, and their physicians are salaried employees. In three of the four examples, these organizations include their own health insurance plans, so that they have complete control of how health care is financed and delivered. Three of these organizations survived major crises in the last ten to twenty years, which doubtlessly influenced the ability of their leadership to implement changes that were often considered radical.

We will not give comprehensive descriptions of these organizations, each of which are worthy of book-length treatments on their own. There are many interesting initiatives under way within these organizations that we will not discuss in this chapter or book. We should also note that these organizations are not the only ones in the United States or elsewhere from which there is much to be learned. The Group Health Cooperative in Seattle, Intermountain Health care in Utah, the Mayo Clinic in Rochester, Minnesota, the Cleveland Clinic in Ohio, and several others could have been used as examples. For the purposes of this book, however, we will focus on one or two key aspects of organized care that these four organizations demonstrate particularly well.

We will begin with the VHA, which has shown how a truly dysfunctional organization can be transformed into a model of reliability for the country—in just a few years, and without a huge infusion of new resources. We will turn to the Virginia Mason Medical Center in Seattle, which has adapted lean management techniques from Toyota to redesign care for patients with back pain and other conditions. Then we will describe Geisinger Health System's innovative CABG program, which offers a glimpse of a new model for paying for health care. And we will conclude with a look at Kaiser Permanente's creative systems to keep populations of patients as healthy as possible.

The VHA: The Turnaround

If the VHA turnaround story has a single lesson for the rest of U.S. health care, it is that even a huge underfunded government bureaucracy can become highly reliable in key areas and much more efficient, if the organization has strong leadership and a mandate to change. The VHA provides care to 5.3 million U.S. military veterans—a population that is older, sicker, and poorer than the general U.S. population. The budget available to the VHA does not increase nearly as much from year to year as medical spending in the rest of the U.S. health care system. Somehow, though, the VHA is managing to set a standard for the country in safety and reliability.

Some readers who have not followed the VHA story may be wondering, "Wait! Are we talking about the same VHA I know about?" Their impressions of the VHA were shaped by movies like the 1992 film

Article 99, which starred Ray Liotta, Kiefer Sutherland, and Forest Whittaker as a group of idealistic physicians struggling to deliver good care despite the insensitive bureaucracy of the VHA. Or they recall the award-winning ABC News special in 1990 that used hidden cameras to capture patient neglect and unsanitary conditions at a VHA hospital in Ohio. These media disasters were in fact reasonable representations of reality. Congressional investigations confirmed that VHA care was deficient in virtually every way, leading to calls to close the VHA down and turn the care of veterans over to the private sector.

Desperate times call for desperate measures, and in 1994, President Bill Clinton appointed Kenneth W. Kizer, MD and MPH, to run the VHA. The former emergency medicine physician and U.S. Navy diver plunged into a seemingly immovable morass with approximately two hundred thousand staff, more than eleven hundred sites of care, and a $22 billion budget. He had to change this unwieldy organization despite resistance from unions and veterans lobbies that were deeply suspicious of any proposals to cut jobs, close facilities, or alter the status quo in any way.

Kizer recognized that he needed to organize the fragmented VHA into regional networks that were accountable for the quality and efficiency of care for large populations of patients—and that had the systems and tools to perform well. His emphasis on the integration and organization of care were clear in testimony that he gave to a congressional subcommittee on July 24, 1997 [1]:

As you know, revolutionary forces are buffeting the entire American health care system. These forces are causing profound changes in private sector health care, as well as in government programs, and they necessitate the creation of new types of delivery organizations. The delivery model being pursued most widely, for a number of reasons, is the integrated service network (ISN)—also known as an integrated delivery system(IDS)—in which organizational entities like hospitals and clinics, partner with physicians and other caregivers, as well as health care support functions, in creative ways to pool their resources and align them to better serve patient needs. These ISNs are taking many forms and are developing in different ways in response to the myriad antecedent conditions and specific circumstances driving their creation. In the veterans health care system, hospital and other facility integrations, as well as clinical and support service integrations, are part of the larger network integration strategy aimed at providing more accessible, reliable and consistently high quality care for as many patients as possible with the resources available.

In this testimony, he went on to describe how the VHA was being reorganized into a series of "VISNs," or Veterans Integrated Service

Networks. He appointed network directors for each VISN, and gave them autonomy to figure out the most efficient way to use their resources. He also gave them enough "cover" from headquarters so that ambitious changes could be made. As he testified, "In the spring of 1995, authority and guidance was issued to the field granting individual medical centers the flexibility to respond to changing local and regional circumstances in the health care marketplace. Organizational changes that add, eliminate, or consolidate clinical and support services at facilities are subject to review and approval by the Network Director. However, proposals to integrate entire treatment facilities under a single management structure are reviewed and approved by VHA Headquarters" [1].

At the time, many members of Congress were unhappy about the consolidation of services within these VISNs that might lead to the closing or downsizing of facilities in their districts. Kizer had already eliminated more than one thousand jobs by consolidating programs. But in the years that followed, those members of Congress would come to applaud the management discipline that was made possible by holding VISN leaders responsible for efficiency and quality in their regions. Management bonuses up to $10,000 were tied to improvement in efficiency, patient access to care, and quality—an early form of pay for performance.

The VISN reorganization started in early 1996, and when Kizer testified before the U.S. Senate Committee on Veterans Affairs on September 22, 1998, he already could describe real progress [2]. He reported that forty-eight hospitals and clinic groups had been merged or were merging into twenty-three locally integrated organizations, and a new capitation system in which the VISNs received fixed budgets expected to be sufficient to care for their populations had been implemented. Among the specific changes he cited were:

• Beginning with about 10 percent of patients enrolled in primary care at the end of 1994, universal primary care has been implemented. By March 1998, 80 percent of the VHA patients surveyed could identify their primary caregiver.

• Between September 1994 and July 1998, more than 50 percent (26,166 of 52,315) of all VHA acute care hospital beds were closed.

• Compared to FY 1994, the annual VHA inpatient admissions in FY 1997 decreased by 24 percent (247,412), while ambulatory care visits increased by 6.6 million (from 25.0 to 32.6 million).

• Between October 1995 and June 1998, the VHA's bed days of care per 1,000 patients decreased by 61 percent (nationally)—from 3,530 to 1,370 (VISN range 980–1,757). This rate is now about 5 percent lower than the projected Medicare rate for the same time period.

• Between December 1994 and April 1998, the VHA's staffing decreased by 11 percent (23,832 of 206,578 full-time employee equivalents), while the number of patients treated per year increased by over 10 percent, including about 8 percent more psychiatric/substance abuse patients, 19 percent more homeless patients, and 21 percent more blind rehabilitation patients.

• Ambulatory surgeries increased from 35 percent of all surgeries performed in September 1995 to about 75 percent in April 1998. Associated with this shift to ambulatory surgery has been increased surgical productivity and reduced mortality.

• Customer service standards have been implemented, customer satisfaction surveys are being routinely performed, and management is being held accountable for improving service satisfaction. Statistically significant improvements have been documented. (In FY 1997, 65 percent of all inpatients—including psychiatric patients—reported the quality of their VHA care as very good or excellent.)

One of the key systems that the VHA was using to improve its care was an EMR known as Vista (Veterans Health Information System and Technology Architecture). An earlier form of Vista was already in evolution when Kizer arrived, but he greatly increased investment in the software along with the training of clinicians on how to use it. Through Vista, complete clinical information is available on any veteran no matter where he or she moves. This advantage was dramatically demonstrated in the wake of Hurricane Katrina, when two VHA hospitals were badly damaged, but their patients were able to receive their care elsewhere without disruption. Physicians receive decision support that guides them to the most efficient medication choice, and reminds them of tests and treatments that are needed by patients with conditions such as diabetes.

The VHA information system does more than capture physician notes, laboratory results, and information on prescriptions. Acting on the suggestion of a VHA nurse, the VHA developed a system for the safe administration of medications. The nurse, Sue Kinnick, had been struck by the efficiency of a car rental agency that used bar codes and scanners to track vehicles and drivers. She convinced administrators at the Eastern Kansas Veterans Affairs Medical Center to use a similar approach to ensure that the correct medications were given to the correct patients [3].

Today, the system suggested by Kinnick is in use throughout the VHA and an increasing number of hospitals in the rest of the country. In this system, nurses wheel small tables with laptop computers linked through a wireless network to the computer system. Before a patient can receive a medication, the nurse waves a bar code scanner over the patient's bracelet and the drug itself to ensure that the right patient is getting the right medication in the right dose at the right time.

The fact that market-changing advances in patient safety should emerge from a health care organization struggling for its financial life might seem surprising at first. But Kizer and other leaders at the VHA knew that they couldn't save it simply by cutting its costs. Thus, the late 1990s was a period during which a wide range of quality measurement and reporting systems were put in place throughout the VHA. An ambitious program to reduce complications for patients undergoing surgery was started, and surgical mortality fell by 9 percent from 1994 to 1998 [3]. That program has now migrated outside the VHA to become a national initiative for improving surgical care [4].

By 1999–2000, a broad range of data began to show the excellence— and even *superiority*—of VHA care. A dynamic young physician leader of the VHA's quality improvement efforts, Jonathan Perlin, MD, reported increases in the proportions of patients who had received mandated immunizations, cancer screening, and counseling for alcohol abuse and smoking that ranged between 130 and 500 percent [5]. Still, the assumption was that care for patients who were really sick in the VHA was inferior to that available elsewhere in the U.S. health care system.

That assumption was challenged dramatically in December 2000, when a young Harvard-trained researcher named Laura Petersen and her colleagues published a study of care for patients with heart attacks (myocardial infarctions) in the *New England Journal of Medicine*. Peterson embarked on the study with the explicit hypothesis that patients sixty-five years old or older who were treated for myocardial infarction in the VHA would receive poorer care and have worse outcomes than patients treated through the Medicare program [6]. They found that patients who were admitted to VHA medical centers had more chronic illnesses and suffered worse heart attacks—yet they had similar death rates at thirty days and one year. In short, the VHA patients were sicker, but they did just as well as non-VHA patients.

The unexpected implication was that VHA care just might be *better* than the rest of the United States. This startling finding began to seem credible after consideration of data showing that the VHA patients with heart attacks were more likely to receive drugs known to reduce complications—beta-blockers, angiotensin converting enzyme inhibitors, and aspirin. VHA patients also were more likely to receive smoking cessation counseling and get good follow-up of their cholesterol treatment by their primary care physicians.

In 2003, even more convincing evidence revealed that something remarkable had happened at the VHA, when data collected by external reviewers showed how quickly VHA care had improved [7]. For example, mammography rates rose from 64 percent in 1994–1995 to 90 percent or more by 1999–2000—versus 77 percent for patients covered by Medicare. For patients with acute myocardial infarction, 95 percent of VHA patients received beta-blockers at discharge, versus 78 percent of Medicare patients. For these and many other important measures, care at the VHA had become more reliable than the rest of the nation.

To be sure, the VHA has had its share of problems. It struggles, as does the rest of the U.S. health care system, with insufficient resources and growing demands. That said, the VHA story shows that major improvement in quality and efficiency is possible within a surprisingly short period—if that care is being supplied by well-organized providers using first-rate systems.

Virginia Mason: Culture Change

In 2000, just as the VHA was beginning to attract attention for its turnaround, the Virginia Mason Medical Center understood that it too needed major change—or that it could very well disappear. This non-profit delivery organization is based around a 336-bed hospital on "Pill Hill" in Seattle, so called because of the nearby presence of several highly respected hospitals. Collectively, these hospitals offer state-of-the-art medical care to Seattle's residents, but also considerable competition to the 400 physicians employed by Virginia Mason.

At the turn of the century, that competition was not going well. Virginia Mason was losing money, and some of its "star" physicians were leaving. Over a period of about five years, however, Virginia

Mason underwent a sweeping change in its culture, enabling it to cut costs, increase revenue, and build a national reputation for quality. The story of how it all began is told and retold at Virginia Mason like folklore.

In 2001, the president of Virginia Mason, J. Michael Rona, was flying home to Seattle, and happened to be seated next to John Black, then the director of lean manufacturing at the Boeing Company. Black had led hundreds of Boeing managers to Japan to study the Toyota Production System, an approach that emphasized constant efforts to eliminate all forms of waste and improve quality. Boeing believed that the impact had been dramatic, and by the time Rona left the plane, he was convinced that Virginia Mason needed to do the same thing.

He found a willing convert in the physician leader of Virginia Mason, Gary Kaplan, MD, who had only recently become its CEO. Kaplan had first come to Virginia Mason in 1978, attracted by the close relationships among its physicians. This culture dated back to Virginia Mason's formation as a physician partnership in 1920 by two doctors who, by remarkable coincidence, both had daughters named Virginia Mason. (Tate Mason's daughter was named Virginia Mason, and his colleague John Blackford had a daughter named Virginia Mason Blackford.)

In 2000, however, Virginia Mason was faring poorly in its competition with nationally known neighbors such as Harborview Medical Center, Swedish Medical Center, and the University of Washington Medical Center. It was losing money for the first time in its history, and staff morale was poor. The administration cut costs, starting with what seemed the least essential. That meant reducing support for research and travel funds that allowed physicians to attend meetings. Some of the better physicians began to wonder if they should stay; others simply left.

Kaplan knew that if Virginia Mason was to survive, it had to change—and the physicians and the management of the delivery organization *had* to collaborate in fundamentally different ways. So work began on developing a formal "Physician Compact": an explicit statement of the obligations of the physicians to Virginia Mason, and what those physicians could expect in return (figure 6.1). The fact that it took more than a year to develop this Physician Compact reveals how foreign the concepts of team care and organization are in U.S. medicine. (Note the logo for "Team Medicine" in the corner of this Virginia Mason summary of its compact.)

Organization's responsibilities	Physician's responsibilities

Organization's responsibilities

Foster excellence

• Recruit and retain superior physicians and staff

• Support career development and professional satisfaction

• Acknowledge contributions to patient care and the organization

• Create opportunities to participate in or support research

Listen and communicate

• Share information regarding strategic intent, organizational priorities, and business decisions

• Offer opportunities for constructive dialogue

• Provide regular, written evaluation and feedback

Educate

• Support and facilitate teaching, GME, and CME

• Provide information and tools necessary to improve practice

Reward

• Provide clear compensation with internal and market consistency, aligned with organizational goals

• Create an environment that supports teams and individuals

Lead

• Manage and lead organization with integrity and accountability

Physician's responsibilities

Focus on patients

• Practice state-of-the-art, quality medicine

• Encourage patient involvement in care and treatment decisions

• Achieve and maintain optimal patient access

• Insist on seamless service

Collaborate on care delivery

• Include staff, physicians, and management on team

• Treat all members with respect

• Demonstrate the highest levels of ethical and professional conduct

• Behave in a manner consistent with group goals

• Participate in or support teaching

Listen and communicate

• Communicate clinical information in a clear, timely manner

• Request information, resources needed to provide care consistent with VM goals

• Provide and accept feedback

Take ownership

• Implement VM-accepted clinical standards of care

• Participate in and support group decisions

• Focus on the economic aspects of our practice

Change

• Embrace innovation and continuous improvement

• Participate in necessary organizational change

Figure 6.1
Virginia Mason Medical Center physician compact. © Virginia Mason Medical Center, 2001 (*Source*: <https://www.virginiamason.org/home/workfiles/HR/Physician Compact.pdf> [accessed December 13, 2008])

As part of its turnaround effort, Virginia Mason had also begun work on a strategic plan, and had reached the conclusion that it had to differentiate itself from its competition. It was not going to perform more or better research than the larger university hospitals nearby, so Virginia Mason decided that it had to distinguish itself through superior quality and by "putting the patient first." But it was uncertain about how it might turn those abstract goals into reality until the concept of Toyota's approach to lean management was introduced to it through Boeing's Black.

"The Toyota Way" is actually a set of five principles defined in 1935 by the company's founder, Sakichi Toyoda. These principles were only formally documented in recent years as the company has employed a

Table 6.1
Five principles of the Toyota way

Continuous improvement	Respect for people
Challenge: We form a long-term vision, meeting challenges with courage and creativity to realize our dreams	*Respect*: We respect others, make every effort to understand each other, take responsibility, and do our best to build mutual trust
Kaizen ("continuous improvement"): We improve our business operations continuously, always driving for innovation and evolution	*Teamwork*: We stimulate personal and professional growth, share the opportunities of development, and maximize individual and team performance
Genchi Genbutsu ("go and see for yourself"): We go to the source to find the facts to make correct decisions, build consensus, and achieve our goals	

growing number of employees outside Japan and recognized the need to train them. The five principles are organized under two "pillars" (see table 6.1) [8].

These principles resonated with Kaplan and Rona, and provided a road map for taking the work under way on the Physician Compact to a functional level. So the next year, they began leading groups of twenty-five to thirty members of their medical center's leadership team to Japan for two-week immersion courses in the Toyota Production System. The message that they gave these leaders—including physicians—was that if they wanted to remain in a leadership role, they must make the physical and cultural journey of this training experience. Not all of them were willing; those who did not are virtually all elsewhere today.

In Japan, these physicians and executives observed assembly lines, and developed their own ideas for improvements that would reduce wasted time, movement, and resources. They helped test their ideas and were thanked by the Japanese when the improvements worked out. They internalized a culture in which improvement goes beyond working in teams on specific projects; instead, waste reduction becomes a way of life. Several reported that the Japanese experience changed the way in which they viewed the world: they found themselves constantly noting inefficiency, and feeling compelled to do what they could to eliminate it.

The authors of this book observed numerous small but telling examples of the depth of this cultural change during a visit to Virginia Mason in 2006. The physician leader who was preparing a conference room for a meeting noted that the projector was stored in a cabinet at the end of the room, far from the one and only place it was ever used (the middle of the conference table). He found himself wondering why it could not be stored on a shelf several feet closer to that spot. Such a change would eliminate just a few seconds of work for people like him who used the conference room. Even though those savings might be trivial, the cumulative effect of constant efforts to reduce waste time, motion, and resources can be significant.

The cultural change at Virginia Mason went beyond a relentless pursuit of efficiency. The leadership of the medical center reached a consensus that it had to be serious about its statement that patients are the most important people in its enterprise. Virtually all physicians and hospitals throughout the world say "Patients come first"—but relatively few are ready to act on the implications of this slogan, which include "Physicians come second."

But Virginia Mason did, with a zeal that caused the departure of some physicians, and occasional grumbling among many who remained. Nevertheless, visitors can see physical evidence of a philosophy that has been summarized as "The Patient Is God" by Chihiro Nakao, a Japanese consultant who advises Virginia Mason. Its new cancer center was designed so that patients would be ushered into well-appointed rooms for the entire duration of each chemotherapy session. There they await the nurses, physicians, and laboratory technicians who come to them. (In most cancer centers, patients do the walking—from the laboratory, to the physician offices, to the chemotherapy infusion rooms.)

The rooms in which the patients sit for their chemotherapy sessions are awash with natural light from large windows. To make that layout possible, physicians work out of relatively small, windowless spaces in the interior of the cancer center. When asked if they mind the new design, one of the physicians paused and then said, "It really is better for the patients." His expression seemed a combination of a grimace and a smile.

The results have drawn nationwide attention. A front-page article in the *Washington Post* in 2005 described the change in the experience of receiving chemotherapy for one longtime patient [9]:

Up until five months ago, Ted Gachowski's weekly chemotherapy appointment was one long, tedious slog through the Virginia Mason Medical Center.

The retired engineer, battling lymphoma since 1999, typically began his journey at 8 a.m. in the first-floor lobby. There he would be directed to the sixth-floor laboratory for blood testing. Next, Gachowski, 63, would board one of the hospital's notoriously slow elevators to meet his oncologist on the second floor. If the lab results weren't ready, he would wait some more. Then back to the elevators for the trek up to 12 and even more waiting. Around lunchtime—if things went smoothly—Gachowski would be seated in a noisy "bullpen" with half a dozen other patients, finally getting the intravenous chemotherapy he came for. By 10 p.m., exhausted from the 17-hour odyssey, Gachowski would arrive home.

Today, chemotherapy at Virginia Mason is a much shorter trip: The distance from lab to exam room to treatment is less than 12 feet. Once Gachowski is hooked up to his IV, he never has to leave the cheery private room—flat-screen television, computer, nursing supplies and bathroom are all right there. And his physician, Henry O. Otero, is so close, "I can almost shout to get him," said Gachowski, seated in a reclining chair as the drug dripped into his arm.

The patient in this *Washington Post* story reported that the changes reduced the time he spent at the hospital by about four hours, saving him energy as well as time. But Virginia Mason also benefits from this streamlined approach. Because patients move through their care processes faster, Virginia Mason increased the number of patients treated per week by about fifty. The increased revenue allows Virginia Mason to hire more staff and support research.

Virginia Mason's transformation and return to financial health have been catalyzed by a combination of visionary leadership and good management skills. Its financial performance in 2007 was its best in the previous five years [10]. Kaplan and his colleagues reassured workers that their efforts to reduce waste would not lead to layoffs. The rank-and-file employees are regularly involved in improvement projects, the results of which are presented each week in a large auditorium to fellow workers and the medical center's leadership. Problems are not swept under the carpet. For example, when a patient died as a result of an anesthesia error, Virginia Mason turned the tragedy into a highly public focal point for its efforts to improve patient safety.

Some visitors to Virginia Mason come away uncertain that a major commitment to a new culture would work in the places from which they came, but almost everyone is impressed that Virginia Mason has figured out how to function like a real organization. The ability of

Virginia Mason to develop an approach to management of lower-back pain that triages patients directly to physical therapy (see chapter 4) is just one case in point [11]. It is also the first medical institution in the country to require all staff to get vaccinated for influenza unless they have an allergy or other condition that makes such vaccination inappropriate. Nationwide, only about one-third of health workers get flu shots; at Virginia Mason, the rate is 98 percent.

Virginia Mason's leaders believe that their cultural change has led to savings in planned capital investment because they are using their space and current buildings more efficiently. They have saved money on inventory, reduced staff walking by thirty-four miles a day, shortened bill collection times, lowered infection rates, and improved patient satisfaction. These changes could not have been accomplished if the hospital, its physicians, and its other personnel had not been forced by crisis into a tight organization with an extraordinary culture.

Geisinger Health System: The Warranty

Around the same time that Virginia Mason was grappling with financial losses and the need for cultural change, another delivery organization on the other side of the country was having an identity crisis of its own: Geisinger Health System was seeking a divorce. In 1996, this northeast Pennsylvania provider organization had merged with the health care providers of Penn State University. This merger was part of a national trend of consolidation among health care providers that was supposed to achieve economies of scale and improve negotiating positions with insurance companies. But the economies had not materialized for this Pennsylvania merger, and the political struggles between the two camps were endless. So the two organizations agreed to part ways in November 1999, less than three years after they had merged. The separation process was completed by June 2000.

Like a divorce for a married couple, this separation was costly to both parties, and Geisinger was left in serious disarray. It "owned" all the components for controlling and delivering excellent health care—an insurance company, hospitals, and a cadre of employed physicians—but the components were not working well together. The longtime CEO of Geisinger stepped aside, and in 2001, an outsider was brought in with a mandate to set things right.

Glenn Steele, MD, was an unconventional choice—a Harvard-trained surgeon who was a key leader at the University of Chicago, but who had little or no prior experience with the health insurance business or managed care, integrated delivery organizations, or rural medicine. But Steele had a reputation as a disciplined manager who could address performance issues, and he was attracted by the potential posed by integrating Geisinger's various components.

Steele changed most of the management team, bringing in several non-Geisinger experts to run the health plan and assume other key leadership positions. The health plan returned to profitability, and some of those funds were (and continue to be) used to support the clinical programs. Investments in the information system were increased, and these systems were used in innovative ways. For example, Geisinger office staff members are given financial incentives to help patients begin using an Internet-based program through which they can access their own laboratory results and communicate with their doctors' offices. Patients not only request a visit through this system but they can also actually book their own appointments and selected tests like mammograms. (Note: one of the authors, TL, is a member of the board of directors of Geisinger Health System.)

Geisinger's use of its information system to improve quality has attracted considerable national attention, but it would be a mistake to limit one's appreciation of Geisinger to its information technology. Steele has sought all along to use software and hardware to coordinate Geisinger's humanware. And the parties being coordinated include patients, physicians, other health care personnel, and the employers paying for the care.

This ambitious vision became explicit in May 2007, when the *New York Times* ran a long front-page story on Geisinger's innovative approach to CABG, opening with the question, "What if medical care came with a ninety-day warranty?" [12]. The article used terms seldom invoked in health care, like "promise" and "guarantee." Geisinger promises that forty important processes will be performed on every elective bypass operation. And while it cannot guarantee a perfect clinical outcome for patients, it does give a warranty of sorts. If patients have any complications related to the operation during the next ninety days, Geisinger provides care at no additional charge.

Skeptics at hospitals around the country, perhaps a bit jealous of the attention Geisinger received after the *New York Times* article, pointed out that most of the specific processes that Geisinger promised to perform were in fact part of routine care. They muttered that Geisinger was swallowing the financial risk of complications in order to pull off a clever marketing ploy.

The truth is that Geisinger has bigger ambitions than drawing attention to its cardiac surgery program. Geisinger's leaders think that their approach—which they are calling ProvenCare—could help introduce a new form of pay for performance for health care providers [13]. And Geisinger believes that tightly structured provider organizations like its own are ideally structured to succeed in such an environment.

The nuts and bolts of Geisinger's new program are far from radical. Geisinger's seven cardiac surgeons agreed on forty processes that should become standard in their care—that is, they should be provided to *every* patient undergoing elective CABG. Most of the "ProvenCare Benchmarks" came directly from guidelines issued jointly by the two major cardiology societies, the American College of Cardiology and the American Heart Association guidelines (see table 6.2) [14]. Many are part of routine care in cardiac surgery departments

Table 6.2
Selected benchmark processes for Geisinger's "ProvenCare" Elective CABG Program

1. Preadmission documentation
- American College of Cardiology/American Heart Association indication for surgery
- Explanation of treatment options to patient
- Is patient current user of clopidogrel or warfarin?
- Screening for stroke risk
- Screening for use of epiaortic echocardiography

2. Operative documentation
- Patient receiving correct dosing of beta-blocker
- Preoperative antibiotics (within 60 minutes of incision; Vancomycin within 120 minutes)
- Use of left internal mammary artery for left anterior descending grafting

3. Postoperative patient documentation
- Antibiotics administered (postoperatively for 24–48 hours)
- Beta-blocker (within 24 hours postoperatively)
- Tobacco screening and counseling

4. Discharge documentation
- Referral to cardiac rehabilitation
- Discharge medications (aspirin, beta-blockers, or statin)

5. Postdischarge documentation
- Patient taking medications correctly?
- Did patient resume smoking?
- Patient enrolled in cardiac rehabilitation?

throughout the country, such as the use of medications like beta-blockers. These standards do not force the surgeons to practice "cookbook medicine," and surrender their judgment and ability to individualize the care of each patient. Yet for each of these forty processes, the physicians must document their reason if they decide a patient does not need them.

There are some items on Geisinger's list of forty that are *not* routine at other hospitals. These additional items reflect the perspective that good quality does not just mean technical excellence; it also means that the surgery truly is needed, the patient understands its risks and wants to undergo the operation despite those risks, and the patient gets follow-up calls after going home to be sure they are on the right track. Geisinger's program requires that surgeons document that patients undergoing CABG have an appropriate reason for surgery according to national guidelines; if they cannot, the case is canceled. The surgeons must also document their discussions of the operation's risks with the patients, and call after hospital discharge to ensure that the patients are taking their medications correctly.

After Geisinger's surgeons agreed on the benchmarks in spring 2006, they looked at a series of cases and found that just 59 percent of the patients had received every one of the processes. In response, the surgical teams began creating systems so that all forty would happen reliably, without disrupting the flow of care. Within a few months, all the patients were receiving all the interventions.

If Geisinger had stopped here, it would probably have improved the quality of its care, but not attracted much attention near its Danville, Pennsylvania, headquarters, let alone the rest of the country. Geisinger, however, was confident enough in its reliability in delivering excellent care that it felt it could go out on a limb financially and offer the equivalent of a warranty for related care within ninety days. For example, there are no additional charges for wound infections or heart failure due to a heart attack that occurs as a complication of the operation. On the other hand, usual charges would apply to care for preexisting heart failure or unrelated problems like a hip fracture.

To come up with its case rate for CABG, Geisinger calculated its historical costs for complications occurring after surgery—and cut them in half. No one knows whether complication rates will really be reduced sufficiently to save this much money, but Geisinger believes that the experience gained by learning how to work within this framework seems worth the risk. Early published data show decreases in hospital use and complication rates [14], and subsequent unpublished data indicate that these favorable trends are continuing.

After the *New York Times* article appeared, large corporations from around the country began calling Geisinger to discuss whether it made sense for them to fly their employees who needed CABG to Danville to get surgery through this program. Geisinger is working on an array of other ProvenCare procedures, including surgery for obesity, cataracts, and major joint disorders. Geisinger is also applying analogous approaches to primary care and the management of chronic diseases such as diabetes.

Whether Geisinger will make or lose money on its case rates is probably not as important a long-term issue as whether health care providers are able to work closely enough together that they can offer something similar to a warranty. (After all, Geisinger can adjust the case rate upward if the costs exceed the revenues.) If this case rate approach becomes something that health insurers and employers demand before they agree to pay top-of-the-market rates to hospitals and physicians, then providers who are not members of groups as well organized as Geisinger will find themselves scrambling to catch up.

Kaiser Permanente: Large-Scale Population Care Excellence

Kaiser Permanente is big—so big that the notion of rolling out a program to improve care across it must seem akin to leading a nation to war. But somehow, this integrated delivery organization that includes a moderately priced insurance plan, dozens of hospitals, and thousands of physicians distributed across the nation has figured out how to do just that. An examination of how it is caring for its patients with diabetes—and saving money at the same time—provides a case study on how a well-organized group of providers can improve care for a population, instead of just one patient at a time.

Founded in 1945, Kaiser is the largest U.S. nonprofit health plan, with nearly nine million members in California, Oregon, Washington, Colorado, Hawaii, Ohio, Virginia, Maryland, Georgia, and Washington, DC. Kaiser includes not only its health plan but also Kaiser Foundation Hospitals and Permanente Medical Groups, which are made up of more than thirteen thousand physicians who are "partners." In truth, Kaiser is made up of several regional organizations that do not always act as one, but throughout the overall organization there are three closely related common core values:

- *Mutual exclusivity* The health plan and medical group are an integrated delivery organization. You cannot have Kaiser insurance without going to Kaiser physicians and hospitals, and Kaiser physicians only see Kaiser patients. If you are a Kaiser patient and go outside the organization for care, you may be responsible for most or all of the costs.

- *Prepayment* The hospitals and physicians function under global capitation; that is, they must provide total care to their populations of patients with the funds collected through the insurance premiums.

- *Multispecialty* The medical groups include primary care as well as specialty physicians, so patients should rarely, if ever, have to go outside Kaiser to receive needed care.

The implications of these core values are profound. Because the care must be delivered within a capped total budget, Kaiser develops systems to prevent medical problems for its patients throughout the year, not just when they are face-to-face with their physicians. In addition, because most patients get virtually all of their care through Kaiser, its systems capture information on virtually everything relevant to patients' care, including what medications they are taking and whether they are actually filling their prescriptions at all. Kaiser is able to remind patients that they need a colonoscopy when they show up at a dermatologist and then schedule the test. Contemplate the likelihood of that happening elsewhere in the U.S. health care system.

As with any enormous organization, there are times when things work, and times when they don't. Kaiser has had well-publicized problems as it has implemented EMRs for its physicians, for example. So has virtually every other large medical group, however, and as of 2008, Kaiser had all of its 8.6 million members receiving routine care with an outpatient EMR, and nearly 2 million members actively used the Kaiser patient portal that gives them access to their records.

When it comes to thinking creatively and then acting effectively to improve the care of populations of patients with chronic diseases like diabetes, Kaiser provides a model that other health care organizations watch closely and try to imitate. Much of the planning of Kaiser's quality improvement efforts occur at its Care Management Institute, which functions like a think tank and change agent for the Kaiser organization. The leaders of the Care Management Institute know that any company of this size would likely turn into a Soviet-style bureaucracy if they tried to dictate the development of programs from their Oakland headquarters. Conversely, Kaiser would not be taking advantage of its structure and systems if its 431 medical offices each charted its own course on key issues. So Kaiser has sought to develop an approach that combines:

• *Local responsibility and creativity*   For example, the responsibility for managing budgets so that the costs of care do not exceed the available resources lies at a regional level. And most of its clinical improvement initiatives begin with pilot projects within one of Kaiser's eight regions.

• *Top-down priority setting*   When a program is believed to have real potential to improve care, Kaiser is able to set goals for the entire organization and create incentives for its regional leaders to reach those goals.

• *Collaboration and shared learning*   Kaiser brings together its physicians and other leaders to facilitate the sharing of best practices and the development of consensus around quality improvement initiatives.

This approach is reflected in Kaiser's program for reducing the risk for heart attacks and strokes for people with diabetes called ALL. Heart attacks and strokes are actually the dominant reasons for hospitalization and death for diabetics, and ALL promotes three highly effective and relatively inexpensive treatments to reduce the rate of these problems. "A" stands for aspirin; "L" stands for Lovastatin, a type of medication called statins that reduces cholesterol levels; and the second "L" stands for Lisinopril, a type of medication called angiotensin-converting enzyme inhibitors that helps protect the kidneys from damage due to diabetes, while also lowering blood pressure. Both Lovastatin and Lisinopril are generic medications, which Kaiser buys at extremely low prices.

The simplicity of ALL is part of its strength. Virtually all the Kaiser physicians (and many nonphysicians) know what the letters stand for and that every diabetic should have at least a trial of each of these three medications. Kaiser physicians know that controlling blood sugar levels for diabetics is important, too, but the fact is that the ALL interventions have much more impact on the outlook for these patients. So ALL dominates the Kaiser diabetes improvement stage.

Outside medical experts who hear about ALL immediately understand its logic and potential impact, but it didn't spring full-blown from Kaiser's clinical leaders. Those leaders describe a time line that looks like this:

- *1990s* Research shows the benefits of various treatments for diabetics

- *2000–2002* Two Kaiser Permanente regions adopt the use of ACE inhibitors for diabetics as quality improvement initiatives, and three Kaiser regions focus on the use of statins for diabetics

- *2002–2003* Detailed analyses of the likely impact of ALL interventions using a sophisticated mathematical model called Archimedes indicate that heart attacks and deaths could be reduced by 71 percent for the 650,000 Kaiser Permanente members with diabetes if ALL was reliably implemented; the expected cost savings were $600 per diabetic per year

- *November 2003* Kaiser's Care Management Institute holds its first ALL conference call to begin planning Kaiser-wide implementation

- *March–October 2004* Regional kickoffs of ALL

The "cycle time" between regional pilots of components of ALL to the nationwide rollout of the full program was just a few years—which might seem long to newcomers to health care, but amazingly quick to those who are currently engaged in such work. Kaiser's leaders are justifiably proud of their speed and effectiveness with ALL, and cite factors including the strong scientific basis behind the ALL interventions, the high priority that the organization's top leadership gave the program, and the ability of local leaders to customize it.

Kaiser is not a one-trick pony that limits its quality improvement efforts to diabetes, of course. Particularly on a regional level, it has implemented impressive programs touching the care of hundreds of thousands of patients. For instance, its northern California region has been working steadily since the early 1990s to reduce mortality for patients with coronary artery disease using a multidisciplinary approach that engages cardiologists, intensivists, emergency department physicians, internists, critical care nurses, and pharmacists in the implementation of guidelines at each of its facilities. Some key interventions include:

- Standing orders and preprinted discharged sheets are used to ensure that patients leaving the hospital are all receiving interventions likely to help them, and are able to understand their care.

- MULTIFIT, an individualized nurse-managed program, lowers the risk for heart attack survivors through lifestyle changes and improved adherence to medications. The first contact between the nurse-manager and the patient occurs while the patient is still in the hospital—a good time for a serious discussion about smoking cessation, proper nutrition, and medications. After the patient goes home, he or she receives scheduled phone calls from the MULTIFIT nurse, and receives written progress reports by mail.

• Patients who decline or have completed MULTIFIT can enroll in Kaiser's Cholesterol Management Program, which helps them reach their appropriate cholesterol goals through phone calls, mailings, and other contact with nurse-managers and pharmacists.

• Kaiser information systems ensure that laboratory results and medication data are readily available to physicians and the nonphysicians who are helping care for these patients.

Kaiser's northern California region can point to a death rate from heart disease for its members that is 30 percent lower than the national average—a result, it believes, of these programs.

Meanwhile, across the country Kaiser's mid-Atlantic states region (covering the Baltimore-Washington-Virginia area) cites a drop in annual asthma hospitalizations for eighteen- to fifty-six-year-olds from 426 in 1999 to 118 in 2004. The tools and tactics are similar to those used in the heart disease program: registries to keep track of patients, analysis of pharmacy claims information to ensure that patients really are taking their medications as instructed, and educational efforts to help patients participate actively in their own care.

Kaiser's Care Management Institute is taking on new and difficult challenges, such as complex patients with multiple chronic problems and the trend toward increasing obesity. The leaders there are also thinking through how an organized group like Kaiser should separate patients into strata so that the complex patients get the most resources, while the worried well get what they need, too. This thinking would be purely academic if it wasn't so critical to Kaiser's business success as a provider organization.

And What about Everyone Else?

The four integrated organizations described in this chapter have nice stories to tell: the VHA's turnaround, Virginia Mason's culture change, Geisinger's guarantees on quality, and Kaiser's effectiveness in improving care for populations of patients. But certain common themes allow them to tell these stories—themes that reflect their tight organizational structures. They employ their physicians. They can make decisions and act on them. They use their information systems effectively. And for those organizations that also own insurance plans, data such as what pharmacy claims are being filled allow them to improve patient care in ways the rest of the U.S. health care system rarely dares to imagine.

As one disease management consultant commented in an article on Kaiser's asthma program,

The Kaiser asthma model could be difficult to replicate in less integrated environments for a number of reasons. ... Kaiser has physicians' attention because it employs them. ... This is not the case in more typical relationships between health plans and community physicians. The more typical case is one in which the health plan and physician have an arms-length relationship. When it comes to physician participation in care or disease management, the health plan has to hope for a collaborative relationship with community-based physicians, but has to rely on carrots, not sticks. [15]

These tight delivery organizations have problems and make missteps, to be sure, but much of the rest of U.S. medicine is so fragmented that simply making a decision that affects more than a handful of hospitals or doctors is impossible. Still, the imperative to make care more efficient and of a higher quality is compelling, and change is under way outside these tight organizations. In the next chapter, we will consider how the organization of care is evolving in the rest of U.S. health care, including our own organization, Partners HealthCare System.

7 Organizing the Mainstream of U.S. Medicine

The organizations profiled in the previous chapter are tightly structured provider groups, which own their own hospitals, employ their own physicians, and often have their own insurance companies. This management structure is sometimes called the clinic model, meaning that all caregivers work for the same clinic, regardless of whether the individuals may be focused on inpatient or outpatient care. When all the components of the provider organization sit under one management team, responding to crises and market imperatives is at least possible—even if collaboration in the improvement of care can be difficult even in these circumstances.

Perhaps advantages derived from this organizational effectiveness will make such tight organizations so attractive to the public that increasing numbers of patients will be attracted to them, and these tightly structured organizations will eventually dominate U.S. health care. The U.S. public seems to value its independence so highly that growth has been sluggish for these "closed systems" within which patients must keep most or all of their care.

For most of the United States, staff model delivery organizations with employed physicians are the exception, not the rule. Can other U.S. providers become organized in ways that bring order to the chaos that characterizes the care received by most Americans? The challenges are formidable. A view from a satellite of U.S. health care would suggest that its main components are academic medical centers, which are built around medical schools and teaching hospitals. This view would be misleading. Closer to the ground, it becomes apparent that most health care in the United States is actually supplied in small physician practices, which generally function like the small businesses they are.

The good news is that these small practices frequently offer wonderful, personalized service to their patients, reflecting the pride of ownership of the physicians who run them. The bad news, as described earlier in this book, is that these small practices are usually not connected to each other or hospitals electronically and in other ways. This isolation reflects the cultural tendency of U.S. physicians to work alone—a tendency that is reinforced by a fee-for-service payment system that rewards doctor visits and hospitalizations, but not patients' overall care.

In this chapter, we will describe two models through which the organization of care can come to this fragmented mainstream of U.S. medicine. The first is a description of our own organization, Partners HealthCare System, which includes two major teaching hospitals as well as community hospitals and more than two thousand nonemployed community physicians. Partners is an example of a provider organization that includes all of the pieces of the tight organizations, but many are semi- or mostly independent, so Partners must work through influence more than control. In this less structured environment, we will look at how Partners is adapting some of the approaches developed by tightly structured delivery organizations. The second is an innovative new approach called the medical home, which proposes bringing systems that organize care into small physician practices— without actually requiring that these physician practices become members of larger organizations.

These are not the only approaches being used to bring organization to the mainstream of U.S. medicine's providers, but they offer a reasonable sense of the strengths and weaknesses of provider-based efforts to improve health care. These insights will be useful in assessing the potential of insurers, employers, and patients themselves to become the organizers of care—topics that will be addressed in the following chapter, and supply the context for considering recommendations in chapter 10 on how providers should change.

The Academic Integrated Delivery System

Like the tightly structured delivery organizations that underwent turnarounds discussed in the last chapter, Partners HealthCare was founded in response to a crisis. In 1994, managed care plans were rapidly increasing their share of the Massachusetts health insurance market and offering hospitals rates that covered marginal but not fully loaded costs. Hospitals had a choice of accepting rates that required a subsidy from other payers or giving up access to a patient population. More often than not, the hospitals capitulated and signed contracts at the lower rates for fear of losing patients.

The managed care plans actually did some real care management, and the length of stay decreased dramatically wherever the hospitals were being paid by the day, while services were shifted to outpatient settings whenever possible. Boston's teaching hospitals found that they were having difficulty with all three of their missions: patient care, teaching, and research. Stand-alone hospitals could not offer the range of care that patients needed, gave medical students only a fleeting glimpse of the sickest patients, and provided a narrow base for medical research. The result was that the traditional academic medical center risked becoming less relevant to its patient community and constituents.

Even against this backdrop, the news that Brigham and Women's Hospital and Massachusetts General Hospital were integrating to form Partners HealthCare System was a shock to the Boston community and much of U.S. medicine. The two hospitals were longtime rivals, both of which enjoyed sterling national reputations. Their training programs for young physicians and researchers were (and remain) among the most selective in the United States. They are both in the *U.S. News and World Report* top ten hospitals virtually every year, while no other city in the United States has more than one on that list.

At each institution, there was tremendous pride, but there was also a reluctance to tinker with traditions that had led to so much success and respect—and to collaborating with counterparts at the other teaching hospital. Their integration was compared by their physicians to the Yankees merging with the Red Sox—an analogy that set off arguments about which hospital was more like which baseball team.

Nevertheless, the senior leadership of the two hospitals understood that change and collaboration were necessary. When Partners Health-Care System was formed in 1994, much of the internal and external attention focused on how the two academic medical centers would integrate with each other [1]. But the more difficult and important challenges have actually been how the academic medical centers would integrate with the providers in the community, and whether Partners would be able to create a true organization that amounted to more than the sum of its components.

This question has been more than an academic issue. Partners Health-Care System is the most prominent provider organization in a market with a high-cost structure for health care and everything else. Besides

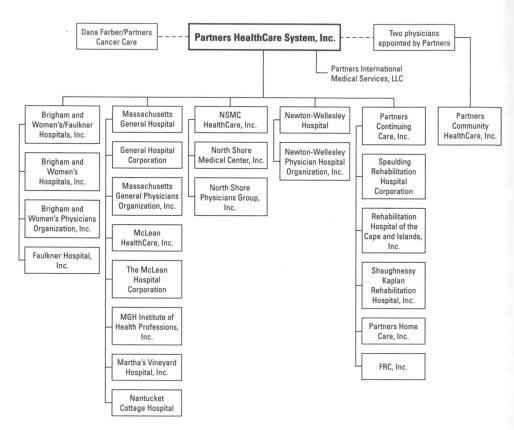

Figure 7.1
Partners corporate organization chart.

its two teaching hospitals, Partners includes six community hospitals, a psychiatric hospital (McLean), three rehabilitation facilities, and about six thousand physicians who deliver care to about two million people (figure 7.1). Even though the market share of Partners is well below that of academic delivery organizations in some other markets, Partners is the focus of considerable public attention at a time of growing concern over rising health care costs.

The question of whether Partners creates value by improving interactions among its hospitals and doctors is especially significant because Partners rejected the bricks-and-mortar strategy that was used in the 1990s by many other academic medical centers. These other institutions bought or merged with other hospitals, and in doing so, often acquired debts, empty beds, and the accompanying problems. Other academic medical centers sought to build a large referral base by purchasing physician practices and making the doctors salaried employees.

Partners wanted to pursue a physician-oriented strategy (as opposed to a facility-oriented bricks-and-mortar strategy), because it believed that physicians ultimately decide where and how care is delivered. But Partners did not want to spend large sums to purchase physician practices. One reason was that the costs would be high. Another reason was that other academic medical centers were reporting that newly salaried community doctors frequently lost the energy of ownership that had previously made their practices successful.

Therefore, Partners built its community network (called Partners Community HealthCare, Inc., or PCHI; see figure 7.1) based on which physicians wanted to work with Partners on contracts with managed care organizations. At that time, Massachusetts health insurance companies were seeking to control health care costs by encouraging physicians to sign contracts for their managed care patients based on capitation (i.e., using a fixed budget to cover all of the health care costs for a defined population of patients). They offered physicians a difficult choice: either the doctors could join groups that signed capitated contracts or they could cease to care for members of that HMO. Because the physicians were concerned about losing access to even a small percentage of their patients, most decided to join groups that were large enough to participate in capitation.

Capitation ran into problems that will be discussed in chapter 11, but one side effect of capitation in Massachusetts in the 1990s was an increase in groupness among providers. Why? First, no one believes that individual physicians should sign contracts based on capitation on their own, thereby taking financial responsibility for their own small population of patients. The incentives to withhold care would be too powerful if every dollar spent came directly out of the physician's income. Capitation requires large patient populations so that the risk of individuals becoming ill (and costly) can be spread over a large group, and it requires providers who are organized enough to adopt systems that might make care more efficient.

With Massachusetts HMOs strongly pushing capitation, physicians in the community began to form independent practice associations or organizations (IPAs or IPOs) and physician-hospital organizations (PHOs) to negotiate these contracts [2]. PHOs are organizations that are jointly owned by a hospital and a subset of the hospital's medical staff members. Most are loosely governed organizations that place a high priority on the inclusiveness of all physicians—often at the expense of improvement in quality or efficiency. IPAs do not include hospitals, and are also loosely governed organizations of multiple physician practices. Because IPAs can be more selective than PHOs about which physician practices are included, though, they have an easier time placing a high priority on performance.

Several of these IPAs, PHOs, and large physician practices concluded that they could get better contracts and help in their efforts to manage care if they joined PCHI. Thus, one of the natural consequences of growing cost pressures in Massachusetts health care was the organization of physicians and hospitals into provider organizations.

Since the mid-1990s, capitation has faded from the Massachusetts health care scene, and been replaced by pay-for-performance programs in which physicians and hospitals get paid on a fee-for-service basis, but have financial incentives to improve quality and efficiency. PCHI contracts include networkwide goals for physicians and hospitals that include improvement in efficiency, quality, and safety (see table 7.1). More than $100 million per year for the physicians and hospitals of Partners is dependent on achieving targets in these areas.

Table 7.1
Partners pay-for-performance goals during 2004–2006

	Physicians	Hospitals
Efficiency	• Reduce medical-surgical hospital admissions • Increase proportion of hospital admissions to community hospitals • Control rate of utilization of high-cost radiology tests • Improve cost-effectiveness of use of pharmaceuticals by outpatients	• Reduce medical-surgical hospital admissions • Increase proportion of hospital admissions to community hospitals • Control rate of utilization of high-cost radiology tests
Quality	• Improve reliability of care for patients with diabetes, asthma, and other chronic disease (NCQA HEDIS measures)	• Improve reliability of care for patients with acute myocardial infarction, heart failure, and other acute illnesses (Joint Commission hospital quality measures)
Information infrastructure	• Encourage use of EMRs	• Adopt CPOE systems

These contracts have therefore provided internal and external pressures to enhance "system value." From the outside, there is pressure from payers and employers on Partners to adopt contract goals and implement systems that help justify its increases in payments. From the inside, there is pressure to develop approaches to ensure that the physicians and hospitals are successful in meeting contract goals, so that the full financial value of the contracts is realized. Collectively, these pressures helped lead to the creation of a Partners' program to reengineer care called High Performance Medicine.

High Performance Medicine

In 2004, Partners launched a program to improve the care delivered in its hospitals and office practices. The program was initially called the Signature Initiatives, and it reflected internally derived ambitions that were reinforced by pay-for-performance contracts and the growing public reporting of data on the quality of care in Massachusetts.

Partners' Signature Initiatives was built around five teams, which collectively constitute a "balanced portfolio" of programs focused on different dimensions of care. This program was renamed High Performance Medicine three years later, and maintains the same team structure (table 7.2) [3, 4]. The first team concentrates on the implementation of EMRs and other information systems with decision support aimed at promoting compliance with guidelines for both inpatient and outpatient care. The remaining four teams build on this clinical information technology base and other systems to improve quality, safety, and cost.

Table 7.3 shows how each of these teams is expected to create value by reducing at least two of the three types of medical errors. Each of these five teams has explicit goals, and their progress is tracked by Partners' CEO (JJM) as well as the boards of directors of the overall system and its individual entities. A color-coding schema (green, yellow, and red) highlights areas that warrant close attention. Progress toward the teams' goals has been integrated into Partners' pay-for-performance contracts. The financial pressures from these contracts add discipline to efforts to reach these targets on schedule.

Collectively, the High Performance Medicine teams have an ambitious agenda that is described internally as constituting two revolutions. The first is an industrial revolution, in which physicians and

Table 7.2
Partners HealthCare System's High Performance Medicine teams

Team	Initial focus	More recent additional focuses
Information technology infrastructure	Deployment of EMRs with decision support throughout community and teaching hospital physician practices	Full and effective use of the EMR
Patient safety	Safe medication prescribing and administration	Reliable transfer of key clinical information as patients move through the healthcare organization
Uniform high quality	Improving the reliability of delivering interventions known to be beneficial for patient populations with diagnoses such as heart failure, acute myocardial infarction, and diabetes	Improving the speed of therapy for patients receiving balloon angioplasty for acute myocardial infarction, and reducing the risk for serious reportable events, including falls leading to injury, infections, and pressure ulcers for hospitalized patients
Disease management	Coordinating care for the most complex and expensive patients	Reducing readmission rates for high-risk patients
Trend management	Developing and implementing guidelines to improve the appropriateness of use of medications and high-cost radiology tests	Reducing unwarranted variation in resource use among physicians

other clinicians adopt tools that enhance quality and efficiency (e.g., EMRs).

The second is a cultural revolution, with several major changes for physicians. Rather than rely on their memories and judgment alone, physicians use decision support embedded in systems like EMRs. Rather than work solely as individuals, they collaborate on teams with other clinicians, particularly in the care of complex patients. And rather than focus solely on the patient in front of them, they take responsibility for populations of patients across continuums of time and places.

Team 1: Information Technology Infrastructure

Hospital and outpatient information systems have the potential to improve the reliability, safety, and efficiency of both inpatient and outpatient care (see chapter 5). Yet the financial and cultural barriers to the

Table 7.3
How Partners' High Performance Medicine teams address the three major types of errors in health care: Examples

Team	Type of errors (see text)		
	Overuse (Inefficiency)	Underuse (suboptimal reliability)	Misuse (suboptimal safety)
1. Information infrastructure	Electronic decision support to guide physicians to cost-effective choices in medications and tests	Systems to identify patients with diabetes who have not received tests and treatments known to improve outcomes	Computerized alerts to prevent patients from receiving medications that might endanger them (e.g., due to interactions with other medications)
2. Patient safety	Systems that prevent medical injuries and thereby reduce costs	N/A	Integrated systems to prevent errors during the ordering and administration of medications
3. Uniform high quality	Highly reliable delivery of optimal care for some subsets of patients (e.g., diabetics), which is expected to improve outcomes and thereby reduce costs	Systems to reliably identify key populations of patients, and ensure that they receive all interventions known to be beneficial	Systems to identify and prevent serious reportable events such as falls that cause injury or pressure ulcers
4. Disease management	Coordination of care to help prevent admission for the highest-risk 3 to 5 percent of patients who account for 50 percent of costs	Team-based programs in which nonphysicians help follow patients to ensure that they are receiving all key treatments	Systems for coordination of care to help identify miscommunication among caregivers that can lead to errors
5. Trend management	Data analyses to identify variation in use of resources; decision support and feedback of data to reduce rate of rise of radiology and pharmacy costs	Development and dissemination of guidelines for appropriate use of medications and tests to increase use for patients who might benefit from them	N/A

Note: N/A = not applicable

implementation of such systems are considerable; thus, a 2005 report estimated that CPOE was in use in about 8 percent of U.S. hospitals with less than three hundred beds, and 17 percent of hospitals with three hundred or more beds [5]. By 2010, these rates are expected to rise to 37 and 53 percent, respectively.

Much of the research demonstrating the potential beneficial impact of CPOE has come out of one of Partners' academic medical centers, Brigham and Women's Hospital. Internal studies indicated that CPOE combined with systems for improving the safety of medical administration has reduced medication errors by as much as 85 percent at Brigham [6]. As a result, the leadership of Partners did not need persuasion that CPOE was a good idea, and Partners achieved full CPOE implementation at its community hospitals as well as its academic medical centers in 2007.

Similar progress has been made in the dissemination of EMRs. At the end of 2003, EMRs were being used by just 9 percent of community primary care physicians in the Partners' network. With the encouragement on incentives built into PCHI's managed care contracts, however, this percentage doubled annually for three years, and about two-thirds of them were using the EMR by the end of 2006 (figure 7.2).

Partners' EMR implementation went well enough so that two unusual decisions were made in 2007. The first decision was about

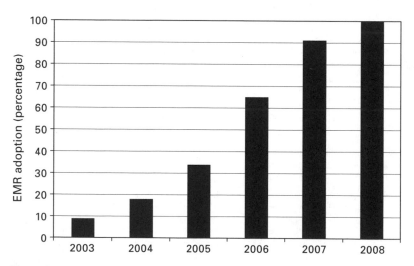

Figure 7.2
Adoption of EMRs by Partners HealthCare System community primary care physicians.

whether to provide direct financial support to physicians to help them implement EMRs. This issue had been moot previously because anti-kickback regulations prohibited hospitals from giving physicians support that could be viewed as an inducement to refer patients to the hospital.

But because the costs of EMRs are so high, federal regulations about what types of financial assistance hospitals could give physicians were relaxed in 2007, so that for the first time, hospitals were allowed to help physicians pay for EMRs. Nevertheless, Partners decided *not* to provide direct financial assistance, because so many physicians had already implemented EMRs that its leadership believed it was past the tipping point. If Partners were to give financial assistance to physicians who were implementing EMRs, it would have to give much of the funding to physicians who were already using EMRs, or risk being accused of rewarding "late adopters" and punishing "early adopters." Instead of using its resources in this way, Partners decided to budget additional resources to improving its EMR and providing additional training in EMR use for physicians.

The second major decision was made by the board of trustees of PCHI, which agreed that the time had come to switch from carrots to sticks in its push toward becoming a network in which all physicians used the EMR. In March 2007, it passed a resolution that *every* primary care physician had to implement an EMR by the end of 2008 or they would be out of the network (and out of its market-leading contracts) as of January 1, 2009. For specialists, similar deadlines were set twelve months later. Press coverage suggests that Partners is the first network in the country with nonemployed physicians to make a policy that actually kicked physicians out if they would not adopt EMRs [7]. Other delivery organizations in Massachusetts began adopting similar policies shortly thereafter.

Having passed the tipping point in EMR adoption, Partners began to turn its attention to the full and effective use of the EMR—especially electronic prescribing. Partners made explicit its goal of having all prescriptions written by computer, so that physicians would be exposed to decision support that would enhance safety and efficiency as they wrote prescriptions, and so that their colleagues would know what medications a patient was supposed to be taking. To turn this aspirational goal into a real-life management focus, Partners negotiated incentives in its pay-for-performance contracts for the percentage of prescriptions being written by computer, and began to profile individual physicians on whether they were prescribing by computer. At some point in the not-so-distant future, Partners expects to make electronic prescribing a requirement for remaining in its network, just as it currently requires the implementation of EMRs.

With the growth of EMR use among community physicians, the reach of Partners' information system increased rapidly. The number of clinical transactions (e.g., prescriptions written, diagnoses entered in problem lists, and notes recorded) increased from ten million in the month of November 2005, to twenty million in the month of November 2006, to thirty million in May 2007. If the work of the other four teams is having the expected impact, these transactions are likely safer, more reliable, and more efficient than they otherwise would be (see next sections).

Team 2: Patient Safety

The second High Performance Medicine team seeks to improve the safety of medication administration—a key focus of the Institute of Medicine reports described in chapter 1. One major goal is to have integrated medication administration systems in place at all Partners' hospitals by 2010 that reduce inpatients medication errors to their lowest possible level. Such systems supplement CPOE systems—which are intended to prevent errors in physician decision making—with systems to ensure that the right patient gets the right drug at the right dose at the right time. As described in chapters 5 and 6, these latter systems include smart pumps as well as an electronic medication administration record that uses bar codes on the medications and patient identification bracelets. Before nurses using this system can give patients their medications, they must use an electronic scan to analyze bar codes on the medication itself and the patient's identification bracelet. Only after the hospitals computer system verifies that, yes, this is the right medication at the right time for this patient, does the nurse go ahead and give the drug.

Research on such systems at one Partners' hospital indicates that CPOE results in a 55 percent reduction in serious medication-related errors [6]. A subsequent study evaluated improvements to the decision support, leading to an 83 percent reduction in the overall rate of medication errors [8]. Other investigations have shown that decision support can reduce rates of complications associated with antibiotics, decrease the rate of hospital-acquired infections and their associated costs [9], and provide evidence for additional benefits from systems that prevent errors during the process of medication administration, such as smart pumps and the bar coding of medications [10].

Still, the number of U.S. hospitals with the complete implementation of such systems is miniscule, with the notable exception of VHA medical centers (see chapter 6). By 2008, such systems were nearly complete at one Partners' facility (Brigham and Women's Hospital) and in progress at the others. And Partners made contractual commitments in its pay-for-performance contracts to have the complete implementation of these systems at all its acute care facilities by 2010. In short, Partners is using its pay-for-performance contracts combined with the high internal profile of its High Performance Medicine program to ensure the management discipline necessary to reach the full implementation of these systems within a few years.

As Partners matures as a delivery organization that takes responsibility for the care of patients in all settings, it has begun to focus on a new issue in patient safety: the challenge of ensuring that key information moves with the patient as they move throughout the delivery organization. In the traditionally fragmented U.S. health care system, doctors do a good job on care that is delivered in their offices, and hospitals do a good job when patients are in the hospital—but neither feels completely responsible for ensuring the accuracy and availability of information like what medications the patient should be taking; when his or her next appointment is, and with whom; what allergies the patient has; and the most recent laboratory test data.

The result is that most patients and physicians have come to *expect* chaos when patients leave the hospital. Patients frequently resume taking the medications that they were on before they were admitted, not realizing that some should be stopped, and others overlap with new drugs started while they were inpatients. Often no one knows exactly what the follow-up plans are for the patient or who to ask.

As more and more of its physicians at its academic medical centers and in the community become online users of its information system, Partners is seeking to realize its opportunity to eliminate this chaos. If a penicillin allergy is diagnosed in a patient seeing a Partners' doctor in New Bedford, which lies fifty miles south of Boston, that information should make it impossible for that patient to receive penicillin if he or she needs to be admitted at Brigham and Women's Hospital or Massachusetts Hospital. And when a patient leaves a Partners' hospital, that patient should leave with key information such as the current list of medications, and how and why his or her preadmission medications were changed.

Most of the U.S. public is surprised that accurate information flow is not a routine part of health care, but to accomplish this goal, Partners had to rewire its information system so that key data elements were pulled together for physicians to review prior to the discharge of the patient from the hospital. Then, to make sure that this review actually occurred, Partners' hospitals instituted a "hard stop"—meaning that it is impossible to let the patient go out the door unless all of the data are available. To make accurate information flow happen reliably as patients move around its system, Partners has had to implement both types of revolutions—industrial and cultural—described earlier.

Team 3: Uniform High Quality

The third initiative seeks to enhance the reliability of the quality of care for key populations of patients, such as those with acute myocardial infarction, heart failure, or diabetes. Crucial functions include the development of software to identify and track populations of patients with diagnoses of interests, the measurement of performance, the comparison of performance to available benchmarks, and the implementation of systems to increase the proportion of patients who receive interventions likely to improve their outcomes.

For example, diabetes is an increasingly common diagnosis for which improved care leads to better patient outcomes as well as cost savings. To improve the reliability of its care, Partners has implemented systems with the functions described in table 7.4. The result has been improvements in the reliability of the care that its diabetic patients receive that have been apparent in public reports on the quality of care as well as the achievement of targets for the improvement in its pay-for-performance contracts. In diabetes and other areas that are the focus of its High Performance Medicine program, Partners uses the nation's ninetieth percentile as its benchmark—and more often than not, exceeds this goal.

More recently, this team has adopted new goals, such as improving the speed of therapy for patients receiving balloon angioplasty for acute myocardial infarction and reducing the risk of falls leading to injury for hospitalized patients. In these and other cases, a common theme has been that performance measures in these areas are or soon will be publicly reported. While Partners' physicians would prefer to

Table 7.4
Systems for improvement of care of patients with diabetes

Function	System
Identification and "tracking" of patient population	Development of computerized registries that can be updated by payer claims data
Decision support software to highlight opportunities to improve care	Electronic records call attention to patients who have not received all recommended interventions, and those whose clinical data (blood pressure, hemoglobin A1c, or cholesterol levels) are not in optimal control
Development of nonphysician clinical team	Diabetes educators (nurses and nutritionists) provide training and continuity of care outside of physician visits
Patient engagement in self-care	Patient educational materials made available to physicians via information system; educational materials sent to homes of consenting patients; support for practices to obtain American Diabetes Association certification (allows for reimbursement for group visits by Medicare)
Financial incentives	Improvement in diabetes care made a major focus of all pay-for-performance contracts
Peer pressure/best practice sharing	Quality improvement forums held at which best practices for diabetes care are shared and recognized with awards

set their own agenda for quality improvement, the fact is that the pressure created by public reporting definitely focuses providers' energy on specific topics. Accordingly, when Partners learns that a new area will be the target of public reporting, this team organizes meetings of Partners' experts, collects and analyzes data, facilitates the sharing of best practices, and tracks progress.

Team 4: Disease Management

The fourth team addresses both quality and cost, focusing on providing highly personalized care for the sickest and most expensive patients. These efforts complement those of the third team, which aims to supply reliable care to large *populations* of patients with specific diagnoses. In contrast, this team uses electronic and other data to systematically identify a small number of high-risk *individuals*, and then connects them to disease management programs that coordinate their care.

These patients tend to have multiple serious conditions such as heart failure, cancer, and depression. They usually receive care from multiple physicians at multiple locations, and are prescribed numerous medications. They are thus the patients who are most vulnerable to errors due to the poor coordination of care. In addition, these patients account for a disproportionate share of costs. They are the 3 to 5 percent of the patients who account for half of all the health care costs.

The potential of disease management programs to improve patient outcomes while also saving costs has been demonstrated most definitively for patients with congestive heart failure. In 1995, Michael Rich, MD, and colleagues reported that a nurse-driven heart failure disease management program could reduce hospital admissions by 56 percent and improve patient quality of life [11]. Relatively few hospitals, however, have implemented such programs because under fee-for-service payment systems, they do not have financial incentives to support programs that prevent admissions.

Through its High Performance Medicine program, Partners funds nurse practitioner–based heart failure disease management programs at its acute care hospitals. Three years of data from this program indicate that it reduces the rates of admission for heart failure for enrolled patients by 15 to 20 percent. At first, the referral of patients to these programs was left to physician discretion, and it quickly became apparent that only about 25 percent of the patients who might benefit from such programs were being referred. Hence, Partners' physician leadership decided that all patients would automatically be referred into the Partners Heart Failure Program or a comparable program unless their physicians indicated that such referrals were not appropriate.

This decision was one of several that reflect a gradual change in culture at Partners in which it is willing to trade some of the autonomy of individual physicians that characterizes the mainstream of U.S. medicine for the effectiveness of the tightly structured delivery organizations described in chapter 6. The leadership of this team recognized that a wonderful intervention (the heart failure disease management program) does not accomplish much good if patients are not referred to it. Hence, a major focus of this team today is ensuring that every patient who is hospitalized with heart failure at a Partners' hospital is evaluated and triaged to a postdischarge disease management program. This task is harder than one might think, in part because the lengths of stay are so short. Partners' hospitals are currently successful in identifying and triaging about 90 percent of the patients with heart failure prior to their discharge.

This High Performance Medicine team developed another program that provides telephonic nurse "coaching" to high-risk Medicaid and uninsured patients. Patients are identified via administrative data, the EMR, and clinician referral. The patients' physicians are contacted by email to seek permission for enrollment in the program. If the physician does not respond within one week, the patient is automatically enrolled, and the call center nurses initiate contact. During any given time, about fifteen hundred patients are actively being coached. Data on the impact of this intervention indicate that it has led to decreases in hospital and emergency department use for these populations, and an improvement in the satisfaction of these patients with the quality of their care.

Team 5: Trend Management

The fifth team directly addresses costs, with programs aimed specifically at mitigating the rise in costs of medications and radiology tests. Decision support systems based on guidelines have been developed to help physicians make cost-effective choices. The recommendations for which medications and tests should be used first are developed by committees of physician experts supported by pharmacists and other staff. The color-coded recommendations are prioritized as green (most favored), yellow (second choice), and red (last choice).

One benefit of these programs for Partners' physicians is related to the increasing use of radiology prior authorization programs by health plans. In such programs, physicians or their staff must call a toll-free number to seek authorization to proceed with a high-cost radiology test such as an MRI or nuclear cardiology scan. Partners' radiology management software has been deemed similar enough in content and likely impact for payers to waive its requirements for such calls by Partners' physicians.

More recently, Partners has turned to a new tactic in its efforts to improve efficiency: showing its physicians how they compare with their colleagues in their use of resources for comparable patient populations. These efforts to address potentially unjustifiable variation require the feedback of data to physicians that show them, for instance, how their use of radiology testing for patients with conditions like lower-back pain compares with that of their colleagues who might be practicing in the room next door.

Physicians at Partners are organized into groups, and these groups are given data on the efficiency and quality of their individual

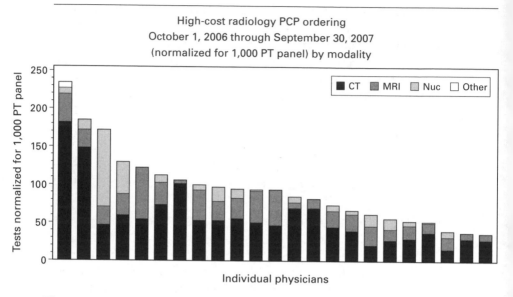

Figure 7.3
Variation among individual physicians in a single practice in high-cost radiology test use.

physicians—and these data are distributed in most groups with the names of each doctor shown. An example of such a report for one physician group is provided in figure 7.3, although the individual doctors' names have been hidden in this illustration. When this report on radiology test use was distributed to the group, the physicians were present in the room, and all of their real names were on this graph.

Ideally, these data should be the start of a process in which doctors give each other feedback, learn from each other, and improve both efficiency and quality (see chapter 10). This program only began in 2007, so the impact of these efforts to improve efficiency by reducing variation remains to be seen. The early results are encouraging, however. In the group of physicians whose data are shown in figure 7.3, for example, radiology test use fell by 15 percent between the first quarter of 2007 and the same time period in 2008.

There is, of course, no gold standard to define success for such efforts to control rising health care costs, as medical progress continues to drive cost increases for patients at Partners and elsewhere. But one measure of success is that Partners' physicians are beating the majority of the targets for efficiency that have been negotiated with payers in its pay-for-performance contracts.

As a result of the progress made at Partners in the first years of its High Performance Medicine program, the targets in its pay-for-performance program have evolved, and are concentrating on new goals that are both more ambitious and more meaningful, such as reducing blood pressure for high-risk patient populations. Such a goal could not have been contemplated without the full implementation of EMRs.

The challenge of implementing these innovations is formidable even for an academic integrated delivery organization such as Partners HealthCare. But how can these systems be implemented in the offices of physicians who are not members of such an organization? In the remainder of this chapter, we turn to an approach that seeks to do exactly that.

The Medical Home

The term medical home is popping up with increasing frequency in the lay press and medical literature. It offers a clear vision of what most people want and what every sick patient needs. The American Academy of Pediatrics writes, "A medical home is not a building, house, or hospital, but rather an approach to providing comprehensive primary care. A medical home is defined as primary care that is accessible, continuous, comprehensive, family centered, coordinated, compassionate, and culturally effective" [12].

If this description is taken seriously in detail, most readers are probably realizing about now that they are medically homeless. For a Commonwealth Fund 2006 Health Care Quality Survey, researchers defined medical homes as regular health care providers who offer timely, well-organized care and enhanced access. These researchers asked respondents whether they had any difficulty contacting their regular providers by telephone or on evenings or weekends, and whether their office visits were generally well organized and running on time. The surveyors found that only 27 percent of adults answered that they had regular providers who met these criteria [13].

Thus, the concept of the medical home is not controversial. The issue is how to help primary care practices evolve so they can provide a medical home to those who want it. An unanswered question is whether the isolated small physician practice that is not part of larger provider organization can take this task on.

What Does a Medical Home Look Like?

The concept of the medical home was developed by U.S. professional societies that represent physicians delivering primary care (the American College of Physicians, the American Academy of Family Physicians, the American Academy of Pediatrics, and the American Osteopathic Association). The basic assumption is that patients are best served if they have direct access to one physician who accepts responsibility for their care, and if that physician practices in an environment that includes systems that are organized to meet all of a patient's medical needs—not just during office visits, but throughout the year, twenty-four hours a day.

On the one hand, the medical home emphasizes a treasured tradition that is now endangered: the primary care physician who knows the patient well, and stands ready to do anything and everything on the patient's behalf. On the other hand, the medical home recognizes that medicine has changed, and that these primary care physicians need to be surrounded by systems like EMRs, and need to lead teams that provide coordinated care and patient education when the patient is not in front of the doctor.

The goals of the medical home are lofty, and are reflected in the Commonwealth Fund's description of seven attributes that should characterize primary care by the year 2020 [14]:

1. Care coordination
2. Clinical information system support
3. Integrated and comprehensive team care
4. Patient engagement
5. Public information on provider performance
6. Routine patient feedback
7. Superb access to care

What are the attributes of a primary care practice that can fulfill this vision? The NCQA's Physician Office Link program is emerging as an approach for deciding which practices meet the standard [15]. (The NCQA's basic function for many years has been reviewing and accrediting HMOs, and it is now adapting its approaches to accrediting physician practices.) The exact criteria that the NCQA uses to certify physician practices are in evolution, but they focus on the practices' ability to pursue these same themes. The NCQA stresses the ability of practices to monitor their patients' medical histories; work with patients over time, not just during office visits; follow up with patients and other providers; manage populations, not just individuals, using evidence-based care; encourage better health habits and the self-management of medical conditions; and avoid medical errors.

Although EMRs are not necessarily an essential characteristic of a medical home, they are definitely part of the vision of virtually all of its advocates. An even more radical change is the integration of non-physician clinicians like nurse educators and care coordinators who are better able to provide the chronic care management and preventive care described in chapter 5. Physicians tend to believe that patients would receive better care if such personnel were part of their practices, as opposed to employees of a disease management company working in a call center that is often in another state. On the other hand, few physician practices have found that it makes business sense for them to hire such staff in a payment system that rewards them primarily for physician office visits.

In summary, a practice that met the criteria of a medical home would be one in which a patient could call (or email) at any time, and get his or her questions answered and needs addressed. The patient's regular physician would take full responsibility for ensuring that the patient's care was well coordinated, and that specialist physicians were communicating with each other and the patient. In between office visits, personnel in the practice would use systems to ensure that all of the patient's preventive care needs were met, and that the patient received the information he or she needed to be the most active participant in his or her own care. In the medical home approach, the primary care physician's practice brings order to the chaos for patients.

How Can Medical Homes Become a Reality?

As attractive as the vision of the medical home may be, the fact is that these homes are costly. They require financial support for physicians to spend time with patients and communicate with other clinicians involved in their patients' care, nonphysician personnel who constitute the teams that work with the patients in between physician visits, and EMRs and other systems that help track the needs of populations of patients over time. The magnitude of these costs and the hoped-for benefits remains uncertain, and will be defined through numerous demonstration projects that are being planned or just getting under way [16].

There are some early tantalizing data from Geisinger Health System and other organizations that there just might be real savings if the medical home is implemented effectively [17]. At Geisinger, one key early finding has been that practices using the medical home arrange primary care physician office visits for most patients within a week or so of discharge from the hospital. This simple step seems to lead to real reductions in the chances that patients get readmitted to the hospital because of complications due to confusion about their correct medication regimens, or a worsening of their condition that can be addressed if detected early.

Medical homes are unlikely to evolve simply by paying primary care physicians more for each office visit. The payment model that is beginning to emerge is one in which physicians get paid standard fee-for-service payments for office visits, but if their practices meet criteria for being a medical home, they receive an additional payment per patient per month. For example, if a health insurer decided to support the medical home model, it would pay accredited physicians some sum for each of its patients who had chosen that doctor as his or her primary care physician (e.g., $3 to $10 per month for patients under age sixty-five, and $30 to $50 per month for older patients, who have higher rates of medical problems) [16]. These funds could be used by the practice to hire a nurse or other staff to handle the care coordination as well as patient education activities that might be expected to improve patients' outcomes.

Some health plans are adding an extra incentive: a percentage of financial savings for the physicians' population, calculated by comparing actual to expected expenditures based on an analysis of their diagnoses. There are usually requirements that the physicians demonstrate high performance on quality measures before they are allowed to share in any calculated savings.

This financial model brings up an inconvenient concern about the medical home: if it truly works, it might only work in larger group practices [18], which are more likely to have systems needed to implement a medical home already [19] and the scale needed to adopt new systems. For example, a nurse care coordinator specializing in high-risk patients tends to carry a caseload of 100 to 125 patients. If these patients represent the sickest 3 percent of all patients, that means those patients have to be drawn from an overall population of 3,000 to 4,000 patients—all from that one insurance company. A typical primary care physician cares for about 2,000 patients, and rarely has more than a few hundred from any one insurance company. Therefore, it is hard to imagine the medical home model with a nurse care coordinator based in the physicians' practice in groups of fewer than 5 to 10 physicians.

For small or even large practices with only a modest number of patients covered under such payment systems, the additional payments that some insurers are offering to support the medical home will not be enough. In such cases, health plans might provide the personnel to perform those educational and coordinating roles, and the physician practice would have to agree to collaborate closely with those health plan personnel. With this approach, the physician practice would not add any personnel but instead receive a small additional per member per month payment for working closely with the health plan's personnel and investing in other systems expected to improve care, such as EMRs.

What percentage of U.S. physicians will make the necessary investments and go through the changes needed to create a medical home for their patients is far from clear. The impact will certainly be quite small if only a few insurers adopt this approach. On the other hand, if Medicare and several major insurers begin offering substantial incentives for practices that meet standards for being a medical home, the proportion of primary care physicians who seek accreditation will rise quickly. The hurdle will be highest for the small physician practices with just one or two physicians, because the ability of these practices to invest in EMRs and hire new personnel is especially limited.

There are relatively few integrated delivery organizations currently seeking to improve their care under pay-for-performance contracts, and those that exist, like Partners, believe that they are far from reaching their potential. And the number of physicians outside these integrated delivery organizations who feel prepared to create medical homes is low.

In the long run, we believe that organizing providers to adopt systems that improve care is the right thing to do. The health care system would probably be more efficient, for example, if it paid a bit more to physicians who used EMRs to help them prescribe the safest and most cost-effective medication. Then it might not have to pay for the companies that analyze pharmacy claims data to detect errors after they have occurred and then try to get physicians' attention to fix them. In other words, it makes sense to cut out the middleperson and reward providers who adopt systems that help them get it right the first time.

But the U.S. health care system is far from ready to reach that goal. So now we turn our attention to what nonproviders can and are doing to bring organization to care.

8 What Can Payers, Employers, and Patients Do?

Although physicians and other health care providers may be best trained and best positioned to bring order to the chaos of modern medicine, most of them are not sufficiently organized to take on this task with optimal effectiveness. Even providers in tightly structured organizations such as those described in chapter 6 frequently fall short of their goals. When providers cannot make care safe, efficient, and reliable, how can the gaps in performance get filled?

In this chapter, we examine the contributions that can be made by payers, employers, and patients themselves. These contributions are aimed in many cases at improving interactions between providers and patients—for example, offering incentives to physicians for helping their diabetic patients control blood sugar and cholesterol levels. The interventions may be aimed at building in safeguards to catch and correct errors, such as disease management programs that detect when diabetic patients have not seen an eye doctor, or to steering patients toward physicians with track records suggesting better performance. In other cases, the interventions do not involve health care providers at all, and try to go around the traditional health care system and improve patients' health directly.

The interventions that involve providers work most effectively when the providers are in well-organized groups. Yet these interventions have been created in part because of the need to improve the care delivered by the fragmented system that dominates U.S. medicine. The U.S. delivery system and the interventions themselves are in active evolution. This final chapter of the first two sections of this book will set the stage for the final section, in which we will examine the issues that will shape that evolution.

Payers

Nature abhors a vacuum—and in the absence of any alternative in U.S. health care, health plans have been the major organizing force since World War II, when employer-sponsored health insurance became a mainstream workplace benefit. Originally, health insurance plans had limited ambitions. They provided protection to members should catastrophic illnesses befall them. To do so, they amassed the funds to pay for physician visits and hospitalizations when patients were acutely ill—and little more.

As costs rose and knowledge of how to *prevent* illness increased, health plans began to struggle with the more complex goals of improving the health of their members and trying to improve efficiency. Both of these tasks are formidable, but U.S. health plans have had both the means and motivation to bring *some* organization of care.

The first of these means are data. Health plans do not know everything that is happening to a patient, but they know about everything that they pay for. The data that the health plans collect as these bills get paid are far from perfect, but they paint a more complete picture of the needs of a population of patients than is available to any other party (see the section on performance reporting below).

The second of these means are the financial resources. Health plans are paid a substantial administrative fee to ensure that their members have access to good health care. These fees tend to range from 8 to 25 percent of the entire health care dollar. With these resources, the health plans decide which doctors and hospitals should be available to the patient, negotiate contracts with those providers, and monitor the quality and efficiency of care. The health plans also use these funds for programs to search for errors (e.g., a diabetic patient who did not get all the recommended interventions).

Finally, health plans have the motivation to organize and improve care. They achieve financial success if they maintain and increase their membership. Growth allows them to spread their fixed costs across a larger population, thereby making the health plans' operations more profitable. How do plans grow? The first strategy is to attract new members by lowering costs—usually by negotiating lower rates with providers, but also by improving the efficiency of care. A more difficult strategy is to improve the quality of care, either by rewarding providers for improved performance or through the use of disease management programs.

In the following sections, we will discuss the three major strategies employed by health plans as they use their control over data and the flow of money to bring organization to health care:

- How they pay providers
- Analysis of data on provider performance
- Implementation of programs that reach around providers, and directly improve quality and efficiency

Paying for Health Care

Payers have the ultimate weapon in health care: they decide what they will pay for, whom they will pay, and how much those providers will get paid (albeit with some negotiation with providers). Health plans have traditionally paid for services performed (fee for service), with the result that they rewarded providers for volume—that is, the number of visits or the number of days spent by patients in the hospital. Although this approach has been adequate for meeting the basic needs of patients who were having an acute illness, it has not directly encouraged a longer-term perspective on patients' health. And the fee-for-service approach has certainly not rewarded efficiency.

Although most U.S. health care is still reimbursed on a fee-for-service basis, a range of other models with greater potential to promote organization and the improvement of care exist. Table 8.1 describes five of the basic approaches, with some comments on the types of providers that can respond to these payment systems—in short, the "receptors" for these "hormones." Hybrids of these models exist, but for the purposes of this discussion, we want to emphasize that the requirement for providers to be organized to respond to the incentives increases as one moves down the list. The relationship between these payment models and the level of provider organization will be discussed further in the next chapter.

If any of these models were ideal for paying for health care, the health care systems of the United States and other countries would rapidly migrate to it. That rapid migration to one model has not occurred, but it is not because the models themselves are inherently flawed. The fact is that these payment models can only be assessed in the context of the level of organization of the providers to which they are being applied.

Table 8.1
Models of payment to providers

Model	Example	Comment
Fee for service	Health plan pays physician $75 for an outpatient visit	Simplest payment approach to administer for fragmented provider organization. Reward for providers to improve quality and efficiency is indirect. Public reporting of quality performance can be used to create competitive pressure for improvement.
Pay for performance	Organized groups of providers receive higher payment if they achieve targets for efficiency and/or quality for the health plan's patients under their care	Growing in prevalence since 2000; data to date demonstrate only modest improvements in quality and efficiency. More organized providers can accept more ambitious targets (see chapter 9).
Case rates	Providers are paid a lump sum for caring for patients during a defined episode of care (e.g., coronary artery bypass surgery)	Requires providers to be organized enough to improve quality throughout an episode of care (see Geisinger ProvenCare CABG description in chapter 6).
Subcapitation	Providers are paid a specific sum per month for meeting patients' needs in defined area of care (e.g., primary care or ophthalmology)	Because appropriateness of providing incentives for efficiency to individual physicians is questionable, this approach requires some organization of physicians. Tends to create tensions among providers, because those receiving subcapitation payments have incentive to off-load work to other providers.
Capitation	Groups of providers are paid a specific sum per month to cover *all* medical needs of a population of patients	Requires highly organized providers with complete or near-complete control over all care patients receive (see description of Kaiser in chapter 6).

For example, when the provider organization is completely fragmented, and most physicians are in one or two physician practices that are independent small businesses, fee for service and tepid versions of pay for performance are about the only models that can be contemplated. These small physician practices tend to respond only to incentives for issues under their control, and they feel only modest influence over the overall costs of care. Health plans can impose incentives on doctors for issues beyond their control, but physicians tend to ignore those incentives except to express bitterness about them.

For this reason, the pay-for-performance incentive programs for the mainstream of U.S. medicine have had only a modest impact on the quality of care and virtually no impact on rising costs. More tightly structured delivery organizations are able to take on more ambitious efficiency and quality goals. These organizations, however, provide care to only a modest percentage of Americans, and pay-for-performance contracts for such organizations only began to evolve about 2000–2001.

Incentives to improve efficiency are inherently problematic for the fragmented mainstream. Most policymakers believe that it would be unethical and poor judgment to offer rewards to individual physicians for controlling the costs of their own panel of patients, since the incentive to withhold care would be too strong. If a physician felt like every additional dollar spent on a patient's care was a dollar out of his or her pocket, the temptation to watch and wait rather than order a test or prescribe a drug would likely work against patients' best interests, even with the most high-minded physicians.

Instead, most policy experts believe, rewards for improving efficiency should be for a large population of patients under the care of a large group of doctors. In that context, physicians can feel peer *pressure* to practice as efficiently as possible, but not experience personal economic fear of the consequences of having a sick or complex patient. We often tell physicians in our own organization, Partners HealthCare System, that we want their goal to be doing everything necessary to meet the needs of the patients in front of them, but we want them to do so using electronic records and other systems such as those described in chapter 5—systems that steer them to the most efficient choices and help them collaborate with their colleagues. This vision is of course impossible without persuading physicians that they should be part of an organized group.

Many policymakers believe that in an ideal world, capitation would be the ideal system of payment. But the vision of that ideal world includes *very* well-organized provider organizations of hospitals and physicians, and it requires that patients receive virtually all their care within those organizations, so that programs to improve efficiency and quality can be fully effective.

Two problems have thus caused many experiments with capitation around the United States to fail. First, U.S. patients place a high value on choice, and do not like being told that they must keep their care within a specific group of physicians and hospitals. And second, capitation has problems dealing with medical progress. Under capitation, health plans have no particular incentive to increase premiums to cover the costs of recent advances.

In truth, *all* systems for financing health care have difficulty accommodating technological progress that leads to increased costs. Capitation is unique in that it shifts the burden for this problem to the providers of care, who tend to be quite unhappy about it. Groups of providers find themselves responsible for managing a budget that might have been adequate for meeting the needs of their patients last year, but is inadequate this year because of the costs of new drugs, tests, and treatments.

A payment system that tends to deny U.S. patients choice and access to progress has two strikes against it. The third strike against capitation has been the fragmentation of U.S. health care—few providers are sufficiently organized to even contemplate signing a contract with capitation as the major method of payment.

But capitation should not be counted out. Some large tightly structured delivery organizations such as those described in chapter 6 are doing reasonably well financially under capitation, and tweaks to the capitation and subcapitation models to make them more broadly viable are being tested. As economic pressures increase in health care, we can expect intense pressure to figure out how to make capitation and the systems for paying providers in the bottom half of table 8.1 work.

In the meantime, health plans also seek to change the market by encouraging patients to *choose* providers that supply better and more efficient care. The most forceful such approach is via "narrowed network" insurance products—for example, a health insurance product in which members can only go to a specific subset of physicians and hospitals. People who sign up for insurance through Kaiser, for instance, must see Kaiser Permanente physicians and go to Kaiser hospitals.

These products allow the health plan to exclude physicians who have a history of generating higher costs for their patients, but their appeal to patients has been limited because of the high value that Americans put on freedom of choice.

Less intense versions of this approach are insurance products with "tiered networks" of providers. In such products, patients can still choose among a wide range of physicians, but they pay more out of pocket if they go see physicians in less favorable tiers. The physicians in the most favorable tier tend to be those with track records of generating lower costs as they care for their patients, while also providing good (or at least adequate) quality of care. These physicians in the more favorable tiers are often in groups that promote quality *and* efficiency. Thus, in theory at least, insurance products featuring tiered networks should move market share to well-organized provider groups—and away from less-organized providers.

Tiered network insurance products are not widespread as yet, however. A major reason is that assessing the efficiency and quality of individual physicians' care requires a great deal of data—and most health plans just don't have enough data to do these analyses for more than a handful of doctors. Physicians placed in less-than-optimal tiers tend to object strenuously to whatever methodology has been used to classify them—and the data and statistical methods that currently exist are quite vulnerable to valid criticism.

Put simply, tiered and narrowed networks are a tremendous hassle for health plans. An easier approach for them is to shift costs to consumers through insurance products with high deductibles (which means patients are responsible for the first portion of health care expenses, such as the first $2,000 of costs generated by their family) or high copayments. In theory, having patients bear more of the financial costs should encourage them to seek out providers that are more efficient and of a higher quality—that is, patients should act more like savvy consumers. And that transformation requires the availability of data on providers, which is the topic of the next section.

Performance Reporting

If knowledge is power, health insurance plans have something approaching a monopoly, since they know about everything for which they have paid. There are, of course, important limits to what health insurance plans know. They do not know about events that do not lead to payments, such as medications that were paid for by the patient using out-of-pocket funds (for example, over-the-counter drugs like aspirin) or prescriptions that were written but never actually filled. And their administrative data do not provide the rich detail of the medical record. For example, it is usually difficult to discern from claims information whether a patient with heart failure has mild, moderate, or severe damage to his or her heart. They also do not know if a clinician calls that heart failure patient at home to make sure that he or she is stable, and not accumulating fluid in his or her lungs, if that phone call is not reimbursed. Hence, the insurance plans' data generally cannot capture the nuances that characterize excellent care.

Nevertheless, health insurance plans have more data than anyone else, with a couple of possible exceptions. Tightly structured delivery organizations (see chapter 6) can capture everything that happens to patients—if those patients receive all of their care from those organizations' doctors, hospitals, pharmacies, and so on. Patients who receive their care from the VHA or a staff model HMO like Kaiser, for example, may face steep financial penalties if they go outside the organization. Therefore, that delivery organization's EMR will have complete information on everything that happened to the patient, with greater accuracy and detail than the administrative claims data available to health plans. The other possible exception is the small percentage of patients who maintain their own personal health records, either in paper files or electronically (see the last section of this chapter).

Health plans have traditionally used their data just for payment transactions (e.g., paying doctors for office visits), but they are increasingly analyzing the performance of physicians as individuals and groups so that the plans can give providers feedback on how they compare with their colleagues, and publish data on which physicians and hospitals appear to perform best on available measures. These published data create a context in which health plans can offer insurance products that include financial incentives for patients to choose providers with better performance (e.g., tiered networks).

There are many knotty issues about how these data are analyzed and used, some of which will be considered in the third section of this book. For the purposes of this chapter, though, it is worth nothing that payers have the ability to analyze their data, and then create financial and nonfinancial incentives to providers and patients (table 8.2). In ideal circumstances, these incentives should stimulate providers to get better organized and offer better care.

Table 8.2
Examples of use of performance data to create incentives for providers and patients to improve care

	Providers	Patients
Financial incentives	Pay-for-performance contracts with greater payments for more efficient/higher-quality care	Insurance products in which patients pay more if they seek care from providers with worse measured efficiency or quality
Nonfinancial incentives	Public reporting of performance data, which creates competitive pressure for improvement for providers	Public reporting, which encourages patients to choose physicians and hospitals with better performance

Several issues have slowed the evolution of that ideal scenario. Thus far at least, patients have shown relatively little interest in the data that health plans publish. In a 2005 survey by Harris Interactive, only about 1 percent of those surveyed reported that they had changed physicians, hospitals, or health plans on the basis of publicly reported data on quality [1]. The tendency of patients to act like consumers and use publicly reported information as they make such choices may increase in the future as patients bear more and more of the costs of their care. But to date, patients have not been attracted to sites that provide performance data on hospitals and physicians.

Providers continue to resist many uses of performance data, citing flaws such as the limited statistical validity of analyses based on the small number of cases on individual physicians, particularly when the analyses are restricted to data available to any one health plan. Providers also complain about the general fallacy of thinking that any one measure of quality or efficiency can describe the performance of a physician, who might be weak in one area of medicine but strong in another. Finally, providers object to being evaluated on the basis of administrative data, which are often inaccurate or unable to capture the severity of illness of patients.

Yet it is difficult to imagine a health care future in which data are not used to measure provider performance and drive improvement. Those analyses will surely be used to create carrots (e.g., financial incentives in pay-for-performance contracts) and sticks (e.g., public humiliation via public reporting or exclusion from insurance products) that will encourage providers to become better organized in the pursuit of improved health care. It seems reasonable to expect that providers will never consider the data and analyses valid enough for the ways they are used. This discontent will be part of the pressure on payers to improve the data and sophistication of the analyses and reporting.

Disease Management Programs

If physicians tend to focus on the needs of the patient directly in front of them, health plans have the ability and motivation to step back, and look at a patient's course over months and even years. They have the data to discern whether a patient is reliably filling his or her prescriptions, and whether his or her physicians have ordered the tests or medications that are known to improve outcomes for chronic conditions such as diabetes. The data are not perfect, of course, and they tend to be a few months behind what is actually happening. Still, health plans have the perspective and resources needed to detect errors of underuse (i.e., instances in which patients have not received what they probably should receive). And the health insurance plans can sometimes step in to try to improve the coordination of a patient's care.

The programs that payers use to bring these types of organization to the care of patients with chronic diseases and complex conditions are often lumped under the label of disease management. Some health plans run their own programs, such as care coordination or case management programs in which nurses help coordinate the care of the sickest and most complex patients. In other cases, as described in chapter 5, health plans contract with companies that specialize in providing disease management programs nationally.

The technical definition of disease management (as per the Disease Management Association of America) is "a system of coordinated health care interventions and communications for populations with conditions in which patient self-care efforts are significant." One implication of this definition is that actions by patients to participate in their own care can make a difference. Another implication is that physicians are not providing sufficient help to patients—and that involvement of physicians may not even be necessary.

Thus, one of the common characteristics of health plan disease management programs is that they tend to carve out the physician and directly interact with the patient. Disease management programs examine claims data to identify patients in the target population—for instance, diabetes. The programs examine data to see if patients are getting everything they should—say, eye examinations. If a patient has not received the recommended intervention, the program contacts the patient, and encourages the patient to contact his or her physician and raise the issue.

There are many variations on this model, but virtually none of the variations depend on direct interactions between the program and physician. After all, communicating with physicians is difficult, and many physicians simply refuse to respond to mail, faxes, or phone calls from these programs. One reason is that physicians are simply over-whelmed with more urgent communications—for example, calls from patients with acute problems that require an immediate response, such as chest pain or fevers. A less lofty reason is that many physicians resent the intrusion of any outside organization into their care for their patients and simply ignore messages from disease management programs.

So disease management programs usually go directly to the patient, via phone, email, or letter. Nurses at call centers interview the highest-risk patients, and sometimes call back on a regular basis to be sure that these patients are stable and have a clear plan for their care. For lower-risk patients with chronic diseases, the programs may simply mail the patient reminders of interventions that they should receive.

These programs are particularly effective when patients have mul-tiple medical problems, or medical problems complicated by social or psychiatric issues—areas that physicians themselves are frequently unprepared to address. For instance, Aetna, a prominent national health plan, enrolls patients with significant medical and behavioral health conditions (e.g., diabetes and depression) in the Medical/Psy-chiatric High Risk Case Management Program. The program's case managers call patients regularly, help them arrange for treatment, provide educational materials, and occasionally contact the patients' doctors with information and reminders (e.g., that the patient needs to be tested for cholesterol levels).

A review of medical, pharmaceutical, and other costs over a one-year period showed some evidence that these patients actually got *more* care than comparable Aetna patients—including higher expenses for medi-cations ($39 per member per month more) [2]. This greater expenditure on drugs presumably reflects encouragement from the program's case managers to the patients to remain on their drugs and take them every day. In addition, the case managers sometimes prompt the patient and/or the doctor to consider adding a drug, such as a beta-blocker for patients with heart failure or coronary artery disease.

The apparent impact of this intensification of care and greater use of medications is lower costs related to hospitalizations and other health care expenses, so that the overall savings from the program is $136 per member per month. The patients in the program also report improvements in their quality of life, and a reduction in limitation at work and in their social life. Some data indicate that patients in these programs miss fewer days from work due to illness.

Does disease management work? On the issue that spawned the disease management industry—that is, the need to control costs—the jury is still out. As noted in chapter 5, a RAND study released in December 2007 concluded that the evidence that these programs save money is soft. On the other hand, there are considerable data that these disease management programs can enhance quality and improve outcomes for patients [3].

Disease management programs are in active evolution, as is true of so much of the health care system. Efforts are under way to enhance their effectiveness through better interactions with health care providers and the patients themselves. Whether these programs will pay for themselves by preventing hospitalizations or even save money remains to be determined. But there is little controversy about the beneficial impact of the longer-term perspective that these programs have brought to the care of patients with chronic diseases and complex conditions.

Employers

Employers' relationships with their employees are complex. The employers want to minimize spending on health care, of course. But they also want to keep their employees happy and healthy, because employers do not like complaints, and they want their workers to be able to show up for work and be productive. They do not want their employees to leave because they are unhappy over their benefits, since the costs of training replacements are high. That said, employees *do* tend to change jobs and move on frequently, so employers have been reluctant to invest in programs that improve health over a long period of time, such as smoking cessation and weight loss initiatives. After all, the chances that the current employer will benefit from better health for the employee down the road are low.

These perspectives are further complicated by the traditional walls between employers and the two key participants in health care: providers and patients. Employees do *not* want their employers to know about their medical issues. And employers generally have not interacted directly with health care providers. There are simply too many doctors and hospitals out there. For their part, health care providers have little interest in spending much time interacting with employers, who do not directly bring them revenue and cannot directly bring them information about their patients.

Because of these walls, employers have looked to health plans to take care of these issues for them. In the fragmented world of U.S. health care, where the focus has been on meeting patients' needs during acute illnesses, what employers have wanted from health plans has been:

• A broad network of physicians and hospitals, so that employees would not complain that they could not see their current doctors

• Negotiated fees for paying doctors and hospitals that were as low as possible

• Reasonable efforts to screen out poor-quality providers

• Programs to improve the quality and coordination of care, such as the disease management programs described in the previous section

Employers certainly still want all these things. Recently, though, larger employers, such as General Electric, Pitney Bowes, EMC, and the agencies that manage employee benefits for some state governments, have sought to take more control of health care quality and costs. These and many other large companies use health plans to do little more than negotiate payment rates with providers and then pay the bills. The companies themselves are exploring options for stimulating the transformation of the health care market to become a more efficient, higher-quality delivery system through financial and non-financial incentives to providers *and* patients. They want to accelerate that transition by encouraging employees to switch to doctors and hospitals that deliver better care, and supporting employees' efforts to take better care of their own health.

Table 8.3 shows some of the major options for employers for driving organization and improvement in health care. The first three types of options are considered variants on the theme of "value-based purchasing." In this approach, employers hope to spend their health care dollars on doctors and hospitals that deliver value—that is, an attractive combination of quality and efficiency. In doing so, employers are indirectly promoting the organization of care, since fragmented providers have difficulty managing either the overall costs or quality of care.

Table 8.3
Employer options for driving organization and improvement in health care

Employer options	Examples
Collecting and reporting data on provider performance	Leapfrog, which reports data on hospital characteristics expected to lead to better patient outcomes
Performance-based provider incentives	Bridges to Excellence, which provides bonuses to physicians whose practices have systems expected to lead to higher quality and efficiency
Insurance products that encourage employees to seek care from providers with lower costs and/or higher quality	Employers can subsidize employee enrollment in tiered network insurance products, or high deductible products that encourage employees to seek care from physicians whose measured performance suggests lower costs and higher quality
Directly implement programs to encourage better employee health	Encourage employees to complete health risk assessments, and use these data to steer employees toward programs designed to improve their health

Two prominent examples of employer-led efforts to transform the health care delivery system are Leapfrog and Bridges to Excellence, both of which were described briefly in chapter 5. These two programs are efforts to drive change in the provider world without directly involving insurance companies, but employers require that health plans be deeply involved in the third option in table 8.3, which seeks to reward higher-quality/lower-cost providers with more market share. These insurance products offer a financial incentive for employees and their families to seek care from physicians whose measured performance indicates greater efficiency and quality.

Thus far, the validity of the data used to classify physicians has been controversial—and even inspired legal challenges from physician societies in New York and Massachusetts. In addition, employees have generally not liked products that shift financial responsibility to them or add complexity to their usual patterns for seeking health care. It is hard for insurance products that are distasteful to patients *and* providers to get very far, but their very existence adds to the pressure on providers to get organized and improve their care.

A relatively new focus among some larger employers is directly working with their employees to encourage better health. These employers still need to keep an appropriate distance from information on individual employees, so they usually work with outside companies like WebMD, which administers confidential health risk assessment questionnaires for employees of many companies. These companies sometimes give employees a financial incentive to complete the questionnaire. The information is used to help direct employees to programs that might improve their health.

Research on workplace-based interventions indicates that these programs can save money, reduce absenteeism, and increase productivity. Some of these efforts have led into areas that have generally been taboo topics for employers, such as mental health. For example, one recent study evaluated a program that identified employees with evidence of depression, using a confidential Web-based and telephone-screening process [4]. Half were assigned to an intervention that included telephone support from a care manager along with their choice of telephone psychotherapy, in-person psychotherapy, or antidepressant medication. The other half received the usual care, which included advice to seek care from their provider.

After a year of follow-up, the participants in the intervention group were 40 percent more likely to have recovered from their depression and 70 percent more likely to remain employed, and had worked an average of two more hours per week than the usual care group. The cost per year of the intervention was $100 to $400, but the estimated value of the additional time worked was far greater.

Employers have also realized that the workplace environment influences the health of their employees. Employers can help people stop smoking by banning smoking on the companies' grounds. And they can help people lose weight by building physical activity into their day.

One major Massachusetts company, for instance, is working with our organization, Partners HealthCare System, to test an approach to helping patients with high blood pressure monitor their blood pressure from their desks at work. Blood pressure measurement devices transmit data via the Internet to Partners, which determines whether the employee's blood pressure is under control, or whether the employee needs to contact his or her physician for a medication adjustment. The expectation is that this approach will allow employees with high blood pressure to achieve better blood pressure control without losing time from work for physician office visits.

Employers are also increasingly aware of the costs and consequences associated with mental health issues. For example, job strain at work has been shown to increase the risk for cardiac complications for employees who have already had a heart attack. One study focused on what happened to 972 people ages thirty-five to fifty-nine who returned to work after heart attacks [5]. All of them underwent extensive interviews about six weeks after returning to work, and then again at two and six years later. "Job strain" was defined by a combination of high psychological demands and low decision latitude. During a follow-up period that averaged about six years, people with high job strain had worse outcomes. Such research has led many employers to develop programs aimed at helping employees deal with job strain and other causes of psychological distress.

Not everyone is going along for this ride, and the reason is of course financial. Smaller companies do not have the resources to take on health care issues; they usually let health plans worry about quality, and just look for the health plan that will do it at the lowest possible costs. And the percentage of large employers who are taking an active approach to changing the health care marketplace through incentives for providers is actually quite low. A 2007 survey of 609 of the largest U.S. employers found that only 16 percent were looking at quality information on physicians, only 2 percent were using the data to reward physician performance, and only 8 percent were trying to influence employee choice of providers [6]. On the other hand, this survey showed that many large employers have developed programs to improve the health of their employees; 83 percent are offering chronic disease management programs, and 70 percent offer health promotion initiatives.

The impact of employer-based health promotion initiatives is far from clear at this point, but there is every reason to believe that they have great potential. After all, working people spend much more time at work than with their physicians. But a growing proportion of Americans are retired, and employer-based programs generally do not help the family members of employees. These gaps raise the question of what patients themselves can do to organize and improve their care.

Patients

Like employers, patients have two fundamental options for improving care. The first is transforming the marketplace, by demanding excellence or moving their business to higher-performing providers. The second is to take control of their own care.

In their effort to transform health care, patients are expressing themselves in a wide range of forums. Consumer organizations have representatives on the major groups that define how the quality of care is measured and reported, including the National Committee for Quality Assurance and the National Quality Forum. A growing number of hospitals and other provider organizations have invited patients to sit on their boards and key committees that oversee the quality of care.

Health plans are surveying patients on their experiences at hospitals and physician practices on a regular basis. These data are often publicly reported and/or used in incentive programs to reward providers whose patients report better service and quality. In general, these patient experience surveys show that patients value physicians who care about them as individuals, remember something about their families, and are readily available when they have needs or questions.

Increasingly, though, patients are interested in systems that go beyond the doctor-patient relationship. Younger patients in particular are attracted to tools that help them to both interact overall with the health care system and take care of themselves. The generations that have become accustomed to ATMs and the Internet want to attend to their business and get their questions answered 24–7—and don't necessarily desire direct contact with a human being in doing so.

To meet this demand, many organized provider groups have been using the Internet to implement "patient portals." Patients can log-on to these secure systems, review their lab data, and ask for appointments, referrals, and prescription renewals. In some organizations, such as Geisinger Health System, patients can actually book their own appointments and mammograms.

Of course, to offer patients this option, providers have to be sufficiently organized that they all use the same scheduling system. And they have to be willing to trust patients as team members who warrant access to the electronic record and scheduling system. Not all physicians are ready to make these leaps. But we expect that in the long run, the physicians who are ready will have a competitive advantage over those who are not.

Finally, some patients want to take complete control of their medical information so that they can be an active "manager" of their care. The motivation for patients to do this is particularly strong when their physicians have not adopted an EMR, or when patients receive care from doctors who are in multiple organizations with records that do not "talk" to each other. An industry is springing up to provide personal health records to this subset of patients.

For example, Microsoft, Google, and other Internet-oriented companies are offering free personal health records on the Web (<http://www.healthvalult.com/>). Microsoft's product, Health Vault, stores, collects, and distributes private health information that can be shared with a physician, a clinic, an emergency department, or a hospital. Information in these personal health records typically includes a patient's medications, list of diagnoses, blood pressures, and laboratory results.

One major concern with these personal health records is privacy. Microsoft and other companies developing these services assure the public that the data will be stored in a secure, encrypted database, with privacy measures that are entirely in the control of the individual. In theory, the patient should be the only person able to determine what information goes in, what comes out, and who sees it.

How will these products be funded? One option is to charge the patient a modest annual fee, but the business model that has worked best on the Internet is to give services away for free and get revenue from advertisers. Therefore, these personal health records will also provide access to information via a search engine, and advertisements are likely to pop up when patients use the site. For example, if someone types "erectile dysfunction" into the search engine, advertisements for medications used to treat this condition may appear.

Microsoft says that its informational searches are strictly anonymous and will not be linked to the personal information within Health Vault. Thus, if one searches for information on sexually transmitted diseases, no record of that search will be stored within the personal health record. Despite these public reassurances, worries about confidentiality persist.

Nevertheless, advocates for personal health records believe that this approach can bring together a patient's health information even if that patient goes to multiple physicians in multiple settings that do not have an integrated information system. When the health care delivery organization cannot provide coordination and continuity, the patient can in theory take charge of his or her data. It is a challenging responsibility, but one that some patients and their families desire and are ready to take on.

III How Do We Get There?

9 Evolution or Revolution?

Change is needed in health care—and change is under way. Physicians and hospitals are implementing systems that make care safer, like EMRs and CPOE systems. With increasing frequency, physicians and nonphysicians are working in teams that coordinate the care of the most complex patients and those with chronic diseases. And retiring physicians are being replaced by a new generation of doctors who are computer savvy and receptive to the notion that being part of an organized team just might be beneficial for their patients.

These changes are being driven by demographic shifts, technological advances, and the demands of an increasingly sophisticated public. The changes are also reinforced by the imperative to deliver state-of-the-art medicine to sick patients. Public report cards provide data to patients and providers themselves on doctors' and hospitals' reliability, safety, and level of service to patients. The systems that we described in chapter 5 and the organization that they imply are increasingly necessary to deliver first-rate care—and no one wants to be revealed as a provider of second-rate health care.

We see these changes playing out in our own organization and in others around the country. The changes require busy physicians to reconsider their culture and learn new skills. These demands cause more than a little stress and unhappiness among our colleagues, but we are sure that the net result is care that is safer, more reliable, and more efficient.

This natural evolution toward a better health care system is encouraging, but are the changes coming quickly enough? For patients and the parties paying for health care, the answer is clearly no. The chaos that we described in the first section of this book is only getting worse, driven by continuing technological progress imposed on our fragmented delivery system. Our rate of organizational improvement is not keeping pace with the need. If there is a race between chaos and organization, chaos is winning.

Although these pressures have been building for decades, a new sense of crisis has emerged. The worldwide financial turmoil that began in fall 2008 has increased the sense that major change is needed urgently to control health care spending. Patients do not understand why their doctors and hospitals cannot remember who they are. Why else would they repeatedly have to fill out registration forms, and list their medications and allergies, even within the walls of a single institution? They are unsettled when confronted with evidence that their physicians are not really in touch with each other. And they are panicked by the increasing financial burdens of paying for their care.

Patients and the organizations paying for health care want a revolution. They are demanding lower health care costs. Many call for insurance premiums to rise no faster than the consumer price index (about 3 percent versus the 9 to 12 percent annual increase in health care premiums most employers have experienced in recent years). They want a health care system that gives patients the care and information that they want, whenever they want it. And they want that better health care system right now.

Evolution or revolution? Steady incremental progress or abrupt drastic change? We think there is a middle road that may be more likely than either extreme to produce the improvement needed in health care delivery.

Why the Capitation Revolution Failed

Calls for change in health care often begin and end with proposals for the transformation of the payment system. Fee-for-service payments reward providers for their volume of services, and we need a delivery system focused on quality and efficiency. To spur the development of that better delivery system, logic would dictate that we need dramatic change in the payment system. Most proposals recommend some form of prospective payment in which providers receive a fixed amount for the care of a patient or group of patients. This fixed budget encourages providers to become more efficient. In theory, that efficiency should be achieved without a loss of quality—or the providers lose patients and go out of business.

Thus, there are two common themes in payment reform proposals. The first is to shift some or all of the responsibility for controlling health care costs to providers. In a prospective payment system, physicians and hospitals pay a price if too many tests are performed or too many high-cost medications are prescribed. The second is to use other levers (direct incentives or market forces such as public reporting) to protect quality. Patients might therefore be protected from excessive frugality by the professionalism of their physicians, augmented by public reporting on quality as well as direct incentives for improvements.

No one really wants to bear financial risk in health care, but prospective payment has many advocates even among providers. After all, physicians and other providers are better trained and better positioned to make decisions about the use of health care resources than insurance companies. If anyone should be able to say "no" to a patient, to say that an MRI is not necessary, it should be the doctor who is facing the patient.

The full-blown version of prospective payment is capitation, in which groups of providers receive fixed amounts of money per member per month for each person who signs up for care with them. Under capitation, providers have virtually all of the responsibility for controlling health care costs—an approach that has been working well at Kaiser, the VHA, and other tightly structured delivery organizations. As described in chapter 6, these delivery organizations have been able to develop programs that save costs *and* improve quality, in part because they can decide how care should be organized and delivered.

Even outside these tight organizations, some provider groups have had good experiences under capitation. Within our own organization, Partners HealthCare System, we have seen groups of physicians with capitated populations arrange nontraditional interventions such as the purchase of air conditioners to help asthmatic patients stay out of the hospital in summertime or a stair lift in a patient's home so that she can stay out of a nursing home. In one instance, a physician group arranged alcohol rehabilitation for a patient's family, because the physician knew that the patient would never stop drinking until those around him did the same.

Those interventions would not have been covered by traditional health insurance. In contrast, capitation can provide resources and incentives that allow physicians to help their patients in creative ways. Doing something unorthodox that helps a patient avoid hospitalization is at *least* as gratifying to physicians as a share of the financial savings that result. In fact, knowing how doctors are creatures of their egos, we think many physicians are motivated *more* strongly by the chance to use their ingenuity on behalf of patients than by financial rewards. Capitation, at its best, can provide both.

Why, then, has this payment approach not taken hold among most health care providers in the United States or elsewhere in the world? In many marketplaces including our own, capitation swept through in the 1990s and then faded away—rejected by patients and providers alike. What went wrong?

Our list of "what killed the 1990s' capitation revolution" in Massachusetts is described below.

• *Many patients didn't like it*   Patients want freedom of choice. When they become sick or are worried that they might be sick, they want the ability to go to the hospital or doctor that they believe is most likely to preserve their health. Providers under capitation, however, have a strong incentive to keep their patients' care within a small network of providers, who are committed to working together to delivering care as efficiently as possible.

Holding financial risk but not having control about how the money is being spent is unnerving for providers, and puts providers in conflict with their patients who want to go outside their organization. In our experience with capitation, we have never seen providers withhold care that a patient needed. But we have seen many instances in which the patient wanted to go to a doctor or hospital in another organization, another city, or even another country, while the physician thought the patient could receive excellent care locally. The resulting tension was unpleasant, to say the least.

• *Many physicians didn't like it*   There are exceptions, of course, and some groups of physicians that collaborate well with each other and their patients have a strong preference for capitation over fee for service. Yet a major problem with capitation has been that many physicians do not like saying "no" to patients or their colleagues, even when it is an appropriate answer. They do not like telling patients that they don't really need the MRI for their headaches or the drugs advertised on television. They do not like telling patients that they should not go elsewhere for their care. And they don't particularly like confronting colleagues who may be less efficient than they could be.

• *Most provider organizations were not big enough*   If a provider group does not have a large number of patients under capitation, it is vulnerable to statistical flukes. A short run of catastrophic luck for their patients—for example, a few new diagnoses of cancer or heart disease—can mean financial disaster for their doctors.

Because the statistical techniques for the adjustment of payments for a population's health risks are far from perfect, capitation can punish physicians for attracting patients with costly conditions like HIV or depression—unless those physicians are part of an organization large enough to have a patient population that is representative of the rest of society. The informal number frequently invoked is a hundred thousand—that is, if you have a hundred thousand people in your population, it is likely to be no sicker or healthier than the rest of the region. It takes a large group of physicians, though, to have this many patients under capitation. If a typical doctor has two hundred patients covered by any one insurance plan, this would mean you must have five hundred primary care doctors in your organization to have a hundred thousand lives.

Few provider organizations have anywhere near this number of doctors and patients. Therefore, physicians working under capitation worry constantly that their patient population might be sicker than average, so that the budget allocated for their care might be insufficient, and there is no completely effective way to resolve those anxieties.

• *Most provider organizations were not effective enough* When we reflect on our own organization's performance under capitation during the 1990s (we lost a great deal of money), we feel that one problem was that we ran out of time. Only recently have most of our physicians begun using EMRs. We were too slow in developing disease management teams to care for patients with conditions like diabetes and heart failure, and when we did organize those teams, they were not as effective as we would have liked. We think we are further along today, and can do a much better job of coordinating care and improving efficiency than in the 1990s. But much of our progress has come a decade too late, and we still have a long way to go.

• *The incentives were not aligned* A basic problem of capitation is that providers are the ones who are responsible for efficiency, but the overall budget (the amount of money available for care) is mainly determined by the health insurance company. The insurer has every incentive to hold down the budget, because lower premiums allow the insurer to attract more members. Provider organizations that negotiate capitated contracts with health insurance plans can push for the highest possible percentage of that insurance premium, but sooner or later, the costs generated by medical progress create an intolerable tension.

Consider, for example, what would happen under capitation if a new drug for diabetes became available—one that did not actually lower patient complication rates but instead was more convenient or had a lower rate of side effects, along with a higher price. Providers would not want to deny the treatment to patients, but insurance companies would be reluctant to increase the budget to pay for it, particularly if the drug did not actually improve patient outcomes. Patients would learn of the drug through direct-to-consumer advertising and then demand it from their physicians. These providers would then argue with the insurers that the budget was not big enough and incur financial losses while the issue was "processed." Meanwhile, the providers would quietly promise themselves that they would never sign another contract under capitation.

That dynamic played out repeatedly in the 1990s, causing the capitation revolution to recede early in this century. Many of the physicians who swore off capitation then are still in practice and have not forgotten their negative experiences.

The Perfect Payment Methodology

In our search for the perfect payment methodology that will support the perfect health care delivery system, two key caveats should be kept in mind. The first is that anytime money changes hands, perverse things can happen. Under fee for service, physicians have an incentive to do more than patients need. Under capitation, physicians have an incentive to withhold care that might be beneficial. These risks are substantially mitigated by the professionalism of physicians, most of whom would be repelled by the notion of subjecting patients to unnecessary risks or failing to offer beneficial care. That said, an important role for policymakers is to recognize the potential dangers created by various payment options and then take steps to minimize them.

The second caveat is that payment systems do not exist in a vacuum. The providers who receive the payments and the patients who receive the services matter. Capitation is an ideal payment system for tightly structured delivery organizations that care for patient populations that cannot go outside of them. The VHA has such a patient population, and people who sign up for care at Kaiser and other staff model HMOs usually know that they are making a commitment to receive their care within that organization. But capitation is more problematic when applied to less-organized providers, especially if they are caring for patients who expect freedom of choice as to which physicians and hospitals they use.

These two caveats lead us to conclude that there is *no* perfect payment methodology for all settings, and that the real search should be for a payment methodology that optimizes the care delivered by the available providers—and nudges them down the road to becoming better in the future.

Figure 9.1, first shown in the introduction of this book, represents schematically a rough relationship between the stages of evolution of providers and the payment methodologies that they can accommodate. On the x-axis, we move from the fragmented world of solo physician

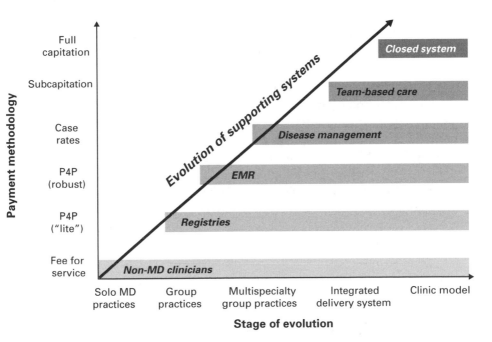

Figure 9.1
Evolving reimbursement and care models. P4P = pay for performance; EMR = electronic medical records. (Reproduced with permission from TH Lee and RA Berenson, "The Organization of Health Care Delivery: A Roadmap for Accelerated Improvement," in *The Health Care Delivery System* [Washington, DC: Center for American Progress, 2008], available at <http://www.americanprogress.org/issues/2008/10/pdf/health_delivery _full.pdf>)

practices to the highly integrated world of tight delivery organizations like Kaiser, the VHA, and Geisinger Health System. In between, physicians become organized into groups. They adopt systems like registries to keep track of their populations of patients. These rudimentary systems need not be electronic. Within our own network, some of the most reliable care in the 1990s was delivered by a group in Brockton, Massachusetts, that kept file cards on its diabetics and other key populations in shoe boxes.

The next succession of leaps for providers requires investment in EMRs, and the development of teams that use nonphysicians to deliver care outside of doctor visits and hospitalizations. Disease management programs coordinate the care of patients with chronic diseases and complex conditions, sometimes with direct involvement from physicians—but sometimes without day-to-day doctor direction. We place our own organization, Partners HealthCare, somewhere in the middle of this progression.

In this figure, payment methodologies are shown on the y-axis. These methodologies range from fee for service to full capitation, in which the providers are responsible for all health care costs. As we have noted in chapter 8, hybrids of these options exist, such as the medical home model described in chapter 7, in which providers are paid with a blend of fee for service and a per member per month payment. Yet the general point that we seek to emphasize is demonstrated by the diagonal arrow going from the lower left to the upper right of this figure. This arrow reflects our belief that more organized groups can accommodate payment methodologies that stress efficiency and quality above the volume of services.

Thus, solo physician practices and small groups are uncomfortable with any payment system besides fee for service. Health insurers can force other incentive structures on physicians in these small organizations, but incentives tend to have little impact when the providers do not believe they can strongly influence their likelihood of success. Indeed, incentive programs with targets that seem unattainable or beyond one's control breed resentment. When providers are sufficiently organized to develop even rudimentary systems, however—like the shoe box registries of our colleagues in Brockton—they can thrive under pay-for-performance incentive programs.

In our figure, we call this early step in payment methodology "pay for performance (lite)" because this type of incentive program is most successful for just one basic type of improvement: reducing the underuse of tests that are likely to be beneficial for the target patient population. Examples of such targets include raising mammography rates for women or improving the rate of cholesterol testing in patients with diabetes. Shoe box registries work fine for this kind of improvement, but fall short for others.

Research has shown that testing cholesterol levels does not necessarily lead to lower cholesterol levels or longer lives for diabetics and other patients. Nor does this lite form of pay for performance foster other types of improvement, such as greater efficiency or improved safety—that is, the decreasing overuse and misuse of care. For a payment methodology to address these more difficult goals, the pay-for-performance models must be robust and the providers need tools like EMRs.

In Partners' pay-for-performance contracts, we now have targets that would have been impossible to consider before EMRs were widespread in our network or before our network was sufficiently organized to take on efficiency goals. Examples of targets in our contracts include:

• Efficiency of pharmaceutical prescribing, which is supported by decision support within EMR prescribing software that guides physicians to the most cost-effective treatment choice

• Efficiency of high-cost radiology test ordering, which is supported by decision support in radiology test ordering software that helps physicians avoid tests that are unlikely to be useful

• Improvement in actual blood pressure, glucose control, and low-density lipoprotein cholesterol levels in patients with diabetes and/or histories of cardiovascular events, which require data that are readily available through EMRs

As we move higher up the progression of payment methodologies, we shift from incentives that have been superimposed on a fee-for-service system to true prospective payment. In true prospective payment methodologies, the financial exposure of the insurance company is limited, and the providers earn something like a dollar for every dollar they save. Of course, the flip side of that coin is that providers are in danger of losing a dollar for every dollar spent unexpectedly.

A good example of case rates was described in chapter 6, in the cardiac surgery case rates offered at Geisinger Health System.

Geisinger guarantees that each elective coronary artery bypass graft surgery will include a preoperative assessment of the appropriateness of the surgery, so that the purchaser can be sure that the surgery was truly needed. And then Geisinger accepts responsibility for providing care for any complication related to surgery that occurs for ninety days after the operation—all for a fixed payment that should represent a savings to the purchaser.

Geisinger hopes to succeed financially under this case rate by improving its quality of care, thereby reducing complications and saving the money that would otherwise be spent addressing them. To improve its quality, provider organizations must do what Geisinger has done—get their clinicians to work together in ways that improve care. Geisinger's cardiac surgery teams all committed to performing 40 key steps that they believe will reduce complications.

It takes a fairly cohesive organization to get clinicians together, get them to agree on what steps are important, and then get them to commit to performing them every time. And because reliable systems *always* involve nondoctors, these teams must include nurses, pharmacists, and other personnel. In short, case rates are impossible without team care.

Subcapitation is a form of prospective payment in which one group of providers accepts prospective payment for the care it delivers, but not for all of health care spending. For example, an organized group of ophthalmologists might accept a fixed per member per month payment for delivering eye care for all of the patients who are enrolled in one insurance plan. The ophthalmologists might accept a lower payment in return for the guarantee that they will receive all of the business from that health plan. The health plan is of course delighted to lock in a lower amount of spending on eye care, but then has to tell all of its members that they can only get eye care from this network of ophthalmologists and also constantly remind other physicians to refer their patients to this network. Under this approach, the ophthalmologists have a strong incentive to develop efficient programs that offer excellent care for the most complex and costly patients—in other words, disease management programs.

Another version of subcapitation is the medical home concept described in chapter 7. In early experiments with the medical home, primary care physicians are often receiving a per member per month payment (along with fee-for-service payments) to supply additional services for their patients. These services include working with nonphysicians to coordinate the care and provide disease management for the patients who are most at risk of requiring hospitalization.

A Warning and a Challenge

Our figure depicts a relationship in which more organized provider groups can work within payment methodologies that involve greater incentives for quality and efficiency—and presumably deliver better and less costly care. We believe that this relationship should help providers and health insurers structure their contractual relationships. The relationships in this figure imply a warning and a challenge, however.

The warning is that payment methodologies should not deviate too far from the diagonal line. Deviations below the line are less dangerous than deviations in the other direction. For example, a tightly structured delivery organization that is engineered to succeed under capitation does not mind taking fee-for-service payments. But if too much of its payment is for traditional fee-for-service care, the tightly organized system no longer has the rewards to support its investment in nonvisit care (e.g., email and telephone contact with patients), disease management, and other programs aimed at keeping patients out of the hospital. A rule of thumb is that prospective payment methodologies need to involve at least 30 percent of a provider group's patients to create a sustained justification for the systems needed to succeed.

Deviations above the line pose a different problem. As highlighted earlier, providers do not like incentives related to issues that they believe are beyond their control or for targets that they do not believe they can achieve. When the payment methodology is above the diagonal line, the provider organization may succeed for a period through luck or extremely hard work, but there is a high risk of failure for the providers. Such failure leads to unhappy providers, and their unhappiness tends to spill over to patients, limiting the durability of payment arrangement.

When there is a mismatch in power in a market such that health insurers can dictate contract terms to providers, you might see ambitious prospective payment systems essentially forced on physicians and hospitals. The 1990s were a time in some markets including Massachusetts in which some health insurers offered only capitation or subcapitation options to many physicians. The alternative for those providers was to forego seeing patients enrolled in those health plans. For a period of a few years, the health insurers did get the providers into contracts based on capitation and subcapitation, but the experience was so dismal that relationships between payers and providers have yet to recover.

The challenge lies in the large diagonal arrow in the figure. The goal of health policymakers and providers should go beyond matching the payment methodology to the degree of organization of the providers. Instead, strategies are needed to move providers to the right—that is, to become more organized, so that they can work successfully within payment methodologies that are more prospective, and will reward better quality and efficiency.

We believe this transformation of health care can occur at a pace faster than evolution, but more successfully than is likely to occur with revolutionary changes, such as imposing capitation on providers who are not sufficiently organized for it. In the remainder of this section of this book, we will describe the needed changes among providers (chapter 10), payment methodologies (chapter 11), and the market itself (chapter 12). These discussions will form the context for our final chapter, which presents our overall prescription for an accelerated evolution to the upper right of our figure.

10   Provider Change

As is probably evident from what we have written thus far, we believe in groupness. We think that the economic challenges and quality issues in health care cannot be addressed effectively unless physicians and other providers are organized into groups that have enough size and effectiveness to adopt tools that improve care. Those tools should help clinicians keep track of data, and make decisions that are safe, efficient, and beneficial for their patients. And these tools should reinforce groupness by helping clinicians work within teams that include patients themselves.

Patients are the real focus of health care, of course, and we think they can bring some organization to care, as can employers and health insurance plans. Nevertheless, perhaps because of where we sit in the health care system, we believe that increasing the organization of providers is the single most critical step needed to meet our health care challenges. If physicians are not organized in groups, they cannot sign contracts with incentives to improve quality and efficiency—one of the most important chicken-and-egg dilemmas that stymie health care. If physicians and hospitals cannot become organized enough to become the targets of incentives for meaningful goals, the incentives have little effect.

The goodness of groupness goes beyond the ability of groups to respond to market forces and adopt systems like EMRs. Larger organizations have visible and sometimes conspicuous roles in society, so they must confront issues that are easily overlooked by small physician practices—issues like care for the uninsured, conflicts of interest, and identification of physicians whose ability to practice has become impaired by mental or other health problems. Larger provider organizations often offer a more orderly life for physicians, so younger doctors today tend to seek employment in larger groups rather than small practices. Because of these demographic trends and the desire of patients for the innovations that larger groups can provide (e.g., Internet connectivity to their medical records), we think organized health care will inevitably "win" over fragmented health care.

There are, however, some bumps in the road between here and there. They cannot be traversed without changes in the payment system and the overall health care marketplace—topics to be addressed in the two chapters that follow. But in this chapter, we focus on changes among health care providers that we believe are necessary to improve care and control costs. Clarity on the goals and barriers to provider change should inform the development of policies intended to hasten the evolution of health care delivery.

We do not believe that the pace of change can be set by demographic trends—that is, we should not just wait for a younger generation of physicians to replace older practitioners. Nor should we expect large numbers of doctors to leap from small physician practices to tightly integrated organizations in which all of the clinicians use the same EMR and work in teams. The disruption to patients and physicians alike would cause unnecessary upheaval. A more realistic expectation is that all health care providers become progressively more organized, making incremental progress down this road regardless of their starting point, adopting tools like EMRs and disease management programs that help them work together along the way.

If more organized health care is better, why aren't physicians and other leaders in medicine moving along this path more quickly? To address these questions, this chapter will describe cultural barriers to change and financial challenges such as the need for capital to fund information systems. We will then turn to a description of some of the skills that health care leaders need to bring greater organization to medicine.

Cultural Barriers

Physician Autonomy

The core of medicine is characterized by altruism, making it a wonderful field in which to work—and a difficult one to change. The goal of health care is to relieve suffering and help people live longer, and the people who are attracted to medicine want to earn their living by doing such work. Physicians in particular train for many years, work long hours, and see themselves as fierce advocates for their patients. For generations, the quality of health care has relied on the high personal standards of the individuals who provide it.

Many laudable aspects of medicine flow directly from these high personal standards, but an unintended side effect can be resistance to increasing organization and collaboration. This apparent paradox begins with the perspective of physicians, who are taught to train all their thoughts and energy on the patient before them.

A tunnel vision outlook is well suited to the work of diagnosis and treatment of disease. Doctors listen to patients' stories, examine their bodies, and review their laboratory tests. They then consider what diseases might explain the findings, which of these diseases are most likely, and which ones have such dire consequences that warrant attention even if they are unlikely. Doctors choose among tests and therapies with different risks and benefits. Sometimes their most difficult choices are the words they use to describe the situation to patients and their families.

It's not easy, this doctor work; it consumes the energy and attention of the intelligent, hardworking people who become physicians. If physicians develop a tunnel vision focus on the needs of the patient before them, they get support for doing so from those very patients. When people are sick or scared, most do not want their physicians thinking about the rising health care costs or the needs of anyone else.

Broad social issues—for instance, the affordability of health care and the improvement of the health of populations through the prevention of disease—are important, of course, but many physicians do not consider these "bigger issues" part of their work. To make vivid the challenge of cultural change for physicians who are focused on the needs of acutely ill patients, we offer the example of one of our colleagues who is known for his brilliance, dedication, and resistance to anything that impinges on his autonomy.

This physician dismisses data that are intended to describe the quality and efficiency of his care. He says that these data cannot capture the needs of his patients, and the nuances of their social and medical problems. He declines (not always politely) to participate on teams, and often refuses to refer his patients to programs in which nurses help follow them between doctor visits. This physician prefers to check on his patients himself.

He is prone to temper tantrums when he feels that others are not doing their jobs, but his patients love him, and his colleagues respect him. They know that when they refer a patient to him, he will not rest until he has done all he can on that patient's behalf. And when other physicians become sick, they often ask him to be their doctor.

This physician is in a one-doctor practice—a small business all his own. He works every day, about seventy to eighty hours per week. He never shuts his beeper off. When his patients are hospitalized, he sees them daily. When his patients come out of an operating room, he is there no matter how late the hour.

He is a hero to many, and a headache to others; he is truly great, but he can be truly grating. Over the years, he has tried working with partners, but those relationships have not endured. He expresses grudging respect for the ideas behind this book, but he was not particularly happy about demands that he adopt an EMR, because it posed a major expense for his practice. Like many physicians, he does not want to be an employee of a large organization that might tell him what to do, even if it might also pay for his electronic record. Although he concedes that in theory, more organization might be the right idea for health care overall, he places an extremely high value on his personal independence, which he believes is critical to the maintenance of his individual standards of excellent patient care.

This physician sees himself as akin to the cowboy—a vanishing breed, not likely to be replaced by younger physicians emerging from their training. He complains that these younger physicians circumscribe their commitments to their work. He points out (critically) that these younger physicians are more likely to turn over the care of hospitalized patients to colleagues who are specially trained in hospital medicine and are in the hospital full time.

These younger physicians are also more inclined to work with non-physicians who can give more time to patient education and provide care outside of doctor office visits. With his heroic efforts, the physician we describe just might exceed what such team care programs can accomplish. But his efforts can be matched by few physicians with young families that need attention, too. To a certain extent, the intense commitment to patients by individual physicians like the one we describe is being replaced by the reliability of teams.

One would like to think that we shouldn't have to choose between passionately dedicated physicians and organized health care. In fact, there are plenty of physicians in effective health care organizations who work just as hard and care for their patients just as intensely as the physician we describe. Yet if we are to argue that team care is absolutely essential to first-rate modern medicine, we should be honest in conceding that team care comes with a price for physicians who treasure their autonomy.

Physicians and everyone else give up some personal independence if they are to be members of reliable teams. They have to trust others to do important work and show respect for them. They have to communicate reliably with others on the team, which means meeting expectations of how they can be reached and what data they will enter in the medical record. As is true of team members in any endeavor, they have to show up for team meetings and learn a playbook. They have to care how their patterns of practice compare with the norms of their peers. We think the sacrifices lead to better care for patients, but the pain of surrendered autonomy is apparent to all who work with physicians.

The Need for Perfection

Physicians' high personal standards of excellence are of course a crucial asset to medicine. These high standards, though, can lead to psychological defense reactions that sometimes actually work against the improvement of care. Physicians are so pained by the implication that they might be making mistakes, that they can be resistant to accepting data demonstrating opportunities for improvement. And because physicians' individual reputations are so important, physicians can be reluctant to confront colleagues who are practicing less efficient or lower-quality medicine unless the evidence of problems is overwhelming.

These two assertions do not sound particularly flattering of physicians, and there are certainly many physicians to whom they do not pertain. Nevertheless, these characteristics are natural themes in a culture where the stakes are so high when a mistake is made. On the one hand, one would hope that the high stakes for patients would mean physicians would have a *low* threshold for accepting data demonstrating problems in the care of their patients or colleagues. But the stakes are also high for doctors' reputations, so physicians often respond to worrisome information by demanding more and more data, and more and more analyses—sometimes making demands that simply cannot be met.

These tendencies are deeply ingrained in the culture of medicine and intertwined with many of the positive features associated with physicians. Because errors can have life-threatening consequences, older generations of physicians (including the authors' cohorts) were taught to rely on no one. Instead, we were trained to check and recheck our own work. This teaching encourages physicians to do their best as individuals, but discourages them from delegating responsibilities to potential team members. It also makes it difficult for physicians to admit that they have made a mistake when one occurs.

After all, the acknowledgment of a mistake threatens physicians' self-image and reputations, and can expose them to malpractice litigation. Thus, recommendations that physicians apologize to patients when they have made errors have elicited a lukewarm response [1, 2]. The very need for such recommendations reflects a culture in which it is difficult to admit to errors.

To be fair, medicine is structured to place the interests of patients ahead of physician egos—and the detection and correction of serious errors is very much part of physicians' lives. About 10 percent of autopsies reveal unsuspected diagnoses [3]; these cases are discussed in medical staff conferences at many hospitals. Surgeons meet regularly to talk about their mistakes and their patients' complications. Physicians who are incompetent or impaired by medical/psychiatric issues are detected and frequently lose their privileges—perhaps not as quickly and reliably as they should, but few nurses or physicians are willing to stand by and let patients be exposed to unnecessary danger.

Nevertheless, the cultural pressure on physicians to never make an error can make it difficult for them to trust others, work in teams, recognize the opportunity for improvement that errors often constitute, or as discussed in the next section, respond to data on their quality and efficiency.

Resistance to Performance Measurement

Doctors are human. In general, they tend to be smart, hardworking humans—but human nonetheless. So when physicians are shown information on their patients that suggests anything less than superlative performance, they often respond by questioning the accuracy of the data or arguing that any deficiencies are not their fault. For example, many doctors become angry when given reports on the percentage of their diabetic patients who not have received eye examinations or the percentage of their diabetics with poor control of their blood sugar levels. They protest that the information is out of date, the list includes patients who are not actually theirs, or their patients are more challenging medically or less reliable than those of other doctors. The patients may not have shown up for scheduled appointments, or failed to comply with their medications or dietary regimens.

Physicians also become upset when shown data suggesting they might be less efficient than their colleagues. They point accusatory fingers at other physicians, who may have ordered many of the tests and treatments that their patients received, and they complain that the patients themselves are demanding expensive drugs and radiology tests. In short, physicians usually believe that they are being evaluated on issues that are beyond their control, using data that are far from perfect.

This anger is understandable, particularly when it comes from physicians whose success in college, medical school, and clinical training was based on excellent performance. And they do have good reason to be leery of "report cards" on their care. The ability of statistical techniques to adjust for socioeconomic status and the degree of sickness of patients is sadly limited, especially when the analyses are based on administrative claims data. Such adjustments may improve as data from EMRs become available for such adjustments. The full use of such information lies far in the future, however, and the ability to adjust statistically for differences among patients will never be completely satisfying.

In addition, most physicians do not have enough patients with any particular diagnosis to provide a valid picture of the quality of their care. Physicians may have several dozen patients with common conditions such as hypertension or diabetes, but for virtually all other diagnoses (e.g., breast cancer, heart failure, or kidney disease), most physicians have too few patients for reliable statistical analyses, unless they are specialists in that area. The result is that report cards on physicians' care can yield wildly varying results from year to year.

The statistical problems of small sample sizes apply to hospitals as well, particularly when dealing with relatively rare events, such as deaths. For example, only about 1 to 2 percent of patients who undergo elective coronary artery bypass graft surgery die. Thus, a typical cardiac surgeon might have just two or three patients per year who do not survive this operation, and a hospital might have only a few more. Mortality rates for cardiac surgeons and hospitals, as a consequence, can be dramatically affected by just one or two deaths.

These deaths might result from the decision to operate on patients with higher-than-average risk or simply from natural variation. For instance, there are five hospitals in Vermont, New Hampshire, and

Maine that share data and collaborate in the care of patients undergoing cardiac surgery. In various years, every one of those hospitals has ranked number one in their death rates, and every one of those hospitals has ranked number five overall. These hospitals have learned that their relative rankings from year to year are not meaningful.

The unreliability of performance measurement is particularly aggravating to doctors when the data are used publicly to rank physicians or hospitals. Cardiac surgeons who are being publicly profiled naturally pause before agreeing to operate on patients with a high risk of complications and death, even if that patient has an even *higher* risk of dying without surgery. Hence, as leaders of a health care provider organization, our position is that data can sometimes be used most effectively for improvement *without* public reporting—by giving the information to providers, acknowledging the weaknesses that may be inherent in the data, and encouraging providers to use the data as the beginning of an exploration of possible opportunities for improvement. Another approach is to publish data on *groups* of physicians, and provide *individual* physician data to those groups so that they can be used in improvement efforts without high stakes of potential public humiliation.

That said, even when data are *not* reported publicly and just used for internal quality improvement, the cultural resistance to data showing room for improvement is a challenge for medicine's leadership. Physicians are so naturally prepared to take responsibility for their patients that it is difficult for them to look at data showing deficiencies as anything other than criticism of them. The truth, of course, is that physicians' panels are merely the organizing unit for the analyses. For example, Dr. Jones's actions are just one of many factors that influence the care of the patients who come to see him. So in theory, he shouldn't be so sensitive when the data suggest a picture that is short of perfection; the data are not really about him.

Then again, Dr. Jones does have *some* influence over what happens to the patients who see him. He chooses the specialists to which his patients are referred, and his patients do listen to his recommendations—even if they do not always follow them. And he does have some say over how his practice functions, such as what happens when patients call with questions or requests, and whether the practice contacts patients who do not show up for visits. So he should not simply ignore data that describe what is happening to his patients.

Confronting Variation

If physicians are *uncomfortable* when confronted with performance data indicating that their patients' care is less than perfect, they are often *confused* when shown data demonstrating variation in their care on issues for which there is no clear right or wrong. Variations in practice patterns among regions and even individual physicians, however, suggest considerable opportunity to improve the efficiency and quality of care [4].

As an example of variation data, consider the percentage of prescriptions written by a physician that are for generic medications. No one wants a physician to prescribe only generic drugs and no brand-name medications. That physician's patients would be missing out on the benefits of recent advances because they would only be receiving older drugs. On the other hand, no physician should prescribe only brand-name drugs, because many of that physician's patients could receive perfectly fine care at lower costs.

So there is no *ideal* percentage of prescriptions that are for generic drugs. Similarly, there is no right rate of use of MRI scans for patients with back pain. And there is no right rate of visits per year for patients with high blood pressure.

Still, there is increasing interest among leaders of health care organizations in showing physicians data on how they compare with their colleagues on such gray zone issues, because substantial opportunities to improve efficiency may lie within them. Physicians make many decisions in the course of a day, and the fact is that for most issues, the right thing to do is unknown. Often, research has not directly addressed the question (e.g., Do patients with high blood pressure have better outcomes if seen four times per year rather than two?). Or if research has been performed, the results are not clearly relevant to the patient at hand—perhaps because the patient is older than those who were in the study or has more complicating medical issues.

In these gray zones, there is tremendous variation in what physicians do. Their decisions are influenced by the behaviors that they have observed in a respected colleague, what happened to the last patient with a similar issue, and their personal willingness to tolerate risk. Compared to their colleagues, some physicians may have a low threshold for admitting patients with chest pain to the hospital, for example, or a low threshold for ordering X-rays. Other physicians may order tests infrequently or send home patients with worrisome symptoms. But without data, physicians do not know how their practice patterns compare with the norms of their colleagues.

Experts on this topic of variation believe that even when there is no clear correct or ideal pattern of practice, it can be useful for physicians to know where they stand compared to other providers. The logic is that if one considers the range of behaviors exhibited by rational and informed people, it might be useful for someone to know if they are at one end of the spectrum or the other, or somewhere in the middle. Figure 10.1 below, for instance, shows rates of head CT scans per one thousand emergency department visits among physicians in the emergency department of a hospital in our organization. There was an eightfold difference in the use of head CT scans between the physician who used the most CT scans versus the physician who used the least. Although there is no clear right answer for how many CT scans per thousand visits these physicians use, in all likelihood there are opportunities for improving the efficiency of care for physicians on the

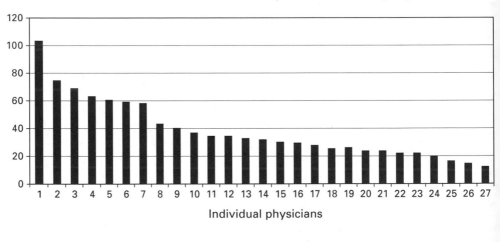

Number of ED CT head exams per 1,000 PT visits per year

Individual physicians

Eightfold variation in rate of use among ED attendings.
Physician 1 uses 40% more head CTs than next highest practitioner.

Figure 10.1
Number of emergency department CT head exams per 1,000 visits per year.

left side of this graph, and there is some risk that the physicians on the right are not using CT scans enough.

In our organization, we provide data to physicians on how their patterns of practice compare to those of their colleagues for syndromes like low back pain and headaches. The reactions range from curiosity to defensiveness. Physicians whose data suggest that they are less efficient than others respond with logical criticisms. They point out that the data are often based on small samples of patients, particularly if the analysis is based on a specific condition, like low back pain. They also note that more resource use might actually be better for patients, and without a comparison of the actual outcomes of patients who receive more or fewer resources, no one should criticize the care of physicians who appear to be "high utilizers." Unfortunately, there are virtually never enough patients, enough data, or enough resources to do that comparison of outcomes, leading some to conclude that variation data cannot provide useful information.

Even physicians who appear to be *more* efficient than their colleagues can be unsettled by data showing that they are low utilizers. After an initial reaction of relief that the data do not suggest that they are inefficient, such physicians sometimes get concerned that they might be giving their patients less care than they should. For example, one of our most respected senior (i.e., over age sixty) physicians received an analysis from a health insurance plan indicating that he used 31 percent fewer overall resources compared to other primary care physicians. He was only partially joking when he commented, "I'm not sure *I* want to go to a doctor who is 31 percent more efficient than other physicians!"

We actually believe that variation data should not be used to classify physicians as efficient or inefficient. The data should be the beginning of an exploration process that focuses on the doctors (or organizations) who appear to be at one extreme or the other. Doctors who use fewer resources than their colleagues might be more experienced, more comfortable with uncertainty, or more out of date than their colleagues. In our organization, we encourage physicians to review each other's charts, so that differences in practice patterns can be identified and discussed.

One of the more gratifying results of such a chart review in our organization came out of an analysis of variations in the care of patients with Hodgkin's disease (a cancer affecting the body's immune system). The ten physicians who specialize in Hodgkin's disease within Partners

HealthCare System reviewed their data and found that they varied widely in their use of an expensive radiology test (PET scan) in their follow up of patients whose Hodgkin's disease was in remission after treatment. In these patients' cases, the goal of care was to monitor patients for any recurrence of disease, so they could be treated as quickly as possible. All of the physicians did regular CT scans, but several of them also performed the much more expensive PET scans once or twice a year.

The physicians reviewed the records of 183 patients and found that the addition of PET scans did not help them identify patients with recurrences any more quickly than CT scans alone. In fact, PET scans incorrectly suggested that recurrences had occurred in twenty-five patients, leading to invasive procedures including the removal of one patient's spleen. The result of the chart review was that the physicians agreed on a new guideline: no more routine PET scans in this type of patient.

In this particular instance, the analysis of the variation data and the subsequent chart review led to consensus among a group of physicians that is saving money *and* improving the care of patients by decreasing the anxiety and risk caused by false positive results. Some skeptics point out that variation data may intimidate physicians at either end of the distribution and cow them into drifting toward the middle of the pack. Quite possibly, no financial savings will result, since low utilizers may increase their use of resources. One of our responses is that analysis of variation data has had a good outcome if efficiency improves among physicians at one end of the distribution and quality improves at the other end. Another is that consideration of variation data should be used as the first step in studies of the patterns of care.

The use of variation data is a relatively new theme in health care, and the best way to pursue this strategy is far from established. Nevertheless, interest in variation data is strong, because of intense concern about rising health care costs. Whatever opportunities to improve quality and efficiency might present themselves through the analysis of variation data, those opportunities cannot be realized if clinicians are unwilling to look at the information and use the data to decide whether to probe deeper into their patterns of care. Our experience suggests that physicians who consider themselves part of an organization are more likely to be willing to undertake this exploration.

Just being part of an organization may not be enough. Research indicates that simply providing information to physicians leads to only modest responses [5]. Variation data may be seen as most useful—and actually get used—when providers have incentives to improve their collective performance [6].

Confronting Colleagues

One last indirect result of physicians' high personal standards of excellence is a cultural aversion to conflict with their colleagues. Physicians pride themselves on the quality of their own care, and they understand that their reputations are critical to their relationships with patients. They also know that damage to the reputations of a colleague can be devastating both professionally and psychologically. With such high stakes, physicians tend to be reluctant to raise criticisms of their colleagues unless the evidence that the other physician is erring is overwhelming.

The result of this form of professional courtesy is health care that is characterized by the individual excellence of smart, hardworking people—but that is limited in the speed and reliability with which it can improve. Even when the evidence strongly suggests that some new approach (e.g., the use of EMRs) improves care, the adoption of that approach is considered optional until the pressures from the external world are overwhelming. Recall the twenty-five years it took for beta-blocker use to become routine for patients with acute myocardial infarction, as described in chapter 4.

When physicians are members of organizations, those organizations can create a context in which physicians are more likely to be evaluated on their quality, safety, and efficiency. A small but meaningful example occurred at one of our hospitals during a campaign to increase hand washing by clinicians before and after seeing patients. As part of this campaign, everyone on the hospital staff was encouraged to confront colleagues who failed to wash their hands—leading to one instance in which a hospital clergyman stopped a physician and pointed out that he appeared to have forgotten this simple act.

In short, the traditional culture of medicine creates a reluctance to confront physicians when their care might be suboptimal. Organizations change that dynamic. In most health care delivery organizations, it is *still* difficult for physicians in particular to criticize other physicians. But the organization of care makes accountability to one's colleagues possible. And organizations of providers can more easily be made accountable than individual physicians to society at large for broader issues, including controlling the rate of rise of health care costs.

Capital: Funding Provider Change

Cultural change is just one of the two key barriers to the organization of providers into groups that can adopt systems that improve care. The second barrier is that systems like EMRs and disease management teams are expensive, and their costs are coming at a time when financial pressures on all segments of the U.S. economy are intense.

The most conspicuous costs associated with our vision of organized care are related to information technology innovations, such as those discussed in chapter 5. These systems include CPOE systems, which reduce errors by physicians as they order tests and drugs, and help identify patients who might benefit from particular interventions (e.g., patients with heart failure or cigarette smokers); electronic medication administration record systems, which ensure that the right patient is getting to right dose of the right drug at the right time; and EMRs for physician offices. The costs of CPOE and electronic medication administration records depend on the size of the hospital, but they can easily reach tens of millions of dollars for an institution. And the cost of EMRs often exceed $10,000 per year per physician (larger physician groups have lower costs per doctor). The start-up costs per physician during the first year are two to five times higher.

These information technology costs are just the tip of the iceberg, and the true costs are frequently higher due to the training required for their implementation and the disruption of well-established work patterns [7]. Sometimes there are cost savings that result from the adoption of information technologies—for instance, fewer personnel are needed to handle paper medical records. Small physician practices, however, often do not have the scale to achieve these savings. For example, if your staff is only one to two people, a reduction in personnel needs related to handling paper records is not likely to make possible a reduction in personnel expenses. Of even greater importance is the general tendency of information technology to improve the *effectiveness* of the workforce in most businesses, but not necessarily to reduce costs. That pattern is definitely apparent in health care.

These information technology expenses are hitting hospitals at a time when other costs are also rising. Medical progress means major new expenses for hospitals. Operating rooms, for example, need to be enlarged to accommodate sophisticated new equipment. New radiology scanners, surgical robots, and the technicians to run them all add millions of dollars to hospitals' budgets.

Personnel costs are also rising, particularly because a national shortage of nurses has led to increases in nurses' salaries well above inflation. About 60 percent of hospital costs are personnel, and about half of those costs are for nursing. Thus, the challenges of holding overall hospital cost increases to the rate of consumer inflation are formidable.

The third major cause for rising hospital costs is the need to deal with problems created by deferred maintenance. During the 1990s, when large HMOs exerted their considerable negotiating power in contract discussions with hospitals, the rates of payment were held virtually flat in many parts of the country. The result was that improvements to the basic infrastructure of hospitals (e.g., lobbies and parking garages) were often delayed. In the last several years, hospitals have sought the resources to make these delayed improvements.

As their expenses are rising, many hospitals and physician practices are losing money on their two largest payers, Medicare and Medicaid. Annual increases in payments from these government payers have been well below increases in providers' costs, reflecting pressure on politicians to avoid tax increases [8, 9]. To make up for this worsening gap, hospitals and physicians have sought higher reimbursement from health insurance plans for commercial populations—a dynamic called cost shifting. The net effect of cost shifting is that insurance premiums for employers increase at an even faster rate than the overall costs of health care, and employers are skeptical about how much longer they can endure annual increases of 8 to 12 percent.

Faced with such increases, purchasers of care are justified in wondering whether they can afford to fund provider adoption of the systems that organize care. Although the potential for provider organization to improve *quality* is obvious, the ability of these systems to reduce overall *costs* is far from certain. Purchasers also worry that when physicians and other providers aggregate into groups, these groups have the ability to negotiate for higher payments.

Some purchasers wonder if their financial interests would be best served if providers did *not* organize themselves, so that contract negotiations would be more one-sided, and health insurance plans could dictate lower payment rates for hospitals and physicians. The logic is that the value of organization and better systems in health care is unproven, and may take years to realize, but the impact of lower prices would be immediate.

Our argument is that this divide-and-conquer strategy implies a short-term perspective. Price reductions extracted from fragmented providers would indeed lead to onetime savings, but the rate of rise due to medical progress and the resulting chaos would continue. Without sufficient resources to modernize their facilities and implement the kinds of systems that can improve care, the chaos would intensify, and our quality, safety, and efficiency problems would worsen.

Skills for the Next Generation of Provider Leaders

To lead physicians and other health care providers into organizations that can bring order to the chaos of modern medicine, leaders need an array of skills that were certainly not part of the medical school curriculum when the authors went to school. Many of these skills are taught in business schools, where an increasing number of physicians and other health care leaders are seeking training either in degree programs or through modular courses lasting several days. But some of these skills *are* being taught at many medical schools today, because educational leaders have learned that no one takes care of patients alone in modern medicine, and working in teams is an important part of being an effective physician.

Strategic Planning

Health care leaders need to develop long-term visions for their organizations—visions that build on potential strengths and are realistic about weaknesses. In the development of these visions, they have to set priorities and make decisions about what they are *not* going to do. They need to develop consensus around these visions, so that they have a chance to succeed in translating them into reality. And they have to understand why transformation efforts so often fail [10].

Unless their organizations are in crisis, the leaders of many health care organizations find the development of consensus around any plan that alienates any constituency difficult—a reflection of the conflict-averse culture of medicine. It is no coincidence that most of the tightly structured organizations described in chapter 6 went through near-death experiences in recent years, without which their leaders would not have had the mandate to push for major change or make difficult choices. For provider organizations that are not in such desperate circumstances, the establishment of a farsighted vision can require especially adroit management skills.

Negotiation and Conflict Resolution

A brilliant plan is worthless unless it can be implemented. To do so, provider leaders must be in constant external and internal negotiations. The external negotiations are with health insurance plans as well as political leaders and employers that collectively represent the purchasing community. These negotiations inevitably include disputes about payment, but also include the development of a shared vision of quality and efficiency goals. The internal negotiations are with the constituents of the provider organization—the physicians and others who must agree to the contract terms, and then work together to meet the goals.

Both types of negotiations can be difficult. Many physicians want to be represented by leaders who will "stick up for us and defend the quality of care"—which can be code for "defend the status quo." Conversely, health care purchasers are understandably preoccupied by immediate financial challenges and are often more focused on constraining cost increases than promoting the evolution of a more organized delivery system.

With both internal and external negotiations, provider leaders need to demonstrate that they understand the needs of their counterparts and propose approaches that address those needs. As political scientists have articulated, negotiation is not really about strength and toughness; it is about understanding and creativity.

Behavioral Economics and Game Theory

These are closely related areas of social science that are particularly useful in negotiation and conflict resolution. Behavioral economics describes rational and irrational patterns in the way people make choices, and can inform the design of incentives. For example, prospect theory, which won the Nobel Prize for Economics in 2002, explains how people put disproportionate emphasis on the risk of small potential losses [11]. This theory suggests that potential losses are a more powerful motivator than potential bonuses. Accordingly, the most effective use of incentive funds is to have multiple targets, each of which leads to a small potential loss if the target is not met. Put simply, it might appear that there is no difference between these two approaches:

• A guaranteed payment of $100, with a potential bonus payment of $20 if a specific quality or efficiency target is reached

• A promised payment of $120, but with the risk that $20 is forfeited if the specific quality or efficiency target is not reached

Prospect theory teaches that the second approach is more likely to produce the desired response.

Game theory was developed by applied mathematicians during the cold war era to help predict likely outcomes when no one individual controls the situation [12]. The classic example of a game is the prisoner's dilemma, in which two separated prisoners must decide whether to "defect" and betray their partner-in-crime. Game theory experiments show that prisoners tend to betray each other in the hope that they will receive more lenient treatment, even though their collective outcome would be better if neither defected.

Although a basic lesson of game theory is that rational but distrusting people have difficulty working together, game theory also provides insight into tactics that increase the likelihood that a collaborative relationship will develop. For example, Robert Axelrod of the University of Michigan has shown that a "tit-for-tat" approach, in which one does *not* ignore aggressive actions by an adversary, leads to collaboration faster and more reliably than "turning the other cheek" [13]. Despite the fact that game theory was developed during the 1950s to model relationships between the United States and the Soviet Union, its lessons are surprisingly relevant to relationships within a health care system struggling to improve.

Process Improvement

A painful reality of the future of U.S. health care is that payments just cannot rise to accommodate increases in costs. Taxpayers are not going to vote for politicians who support even inflationary increases in payments to doctors and hospitals for Medicare and Medicaid patients. And commercial health insurance plans are unwilling to raise their payments to cover provider losses from these government populations.

This dynamic means that health care providers—especially hospitals—must figure out how to reduce their costs. Many other industries, particularly manufacturing industries, have been living with such pressures for decades, of course. While taking care of patients is not like making an automobile, there are lessons to be learned from Toyota and other non-health care companies about how to bring discipline to the quest for efficiency [14].

Virginia Mason Medical Center in Seattle has drawn the most attention nationally for its adoption of the Toyota lean management approach (see chapter 6). Because of the cost conundrum described above, many other health care organizations including our own are also pursuing process improvement programs in which they study their key processes, and try to figure out how to perform them with less wasted time and resources. The analysis of variation data as discussed earlier in this chapter is just one form of process improvement that would be familiar to lean management proponents from other industries.

Systems Theory

Systems theory is a loosely used term that describes interdisciplinary studies of complex systems in nature, society, and biology [15]. It becomes relevant to the organization of health care as the network of health care providers who collaborate in the care of complex patients becomes bigger and broader.

One example of a "system-level" challenge that has emerged for Partners HealthCare System is the question of what functions make the whole greater than the sum of our parts. One such function might be ensuring the reliability of the flow of information across our network of providers. If this function is performed reliably, a patient who is known to be allergic to penicillin by his or her physician in New Bedford, Massachusetts, will not receive penicillin if admitted to one of our hospitals in Boston. And when patients leave our Boston hospitals, their exact medical regimens should be conveyed to their doctors and the patients themselves. This flow of information does not show up as a measure of quality for the doctor in New Bedford or the hospital in Boston, yet it has real value for patients.

Another system-level challenge is social network analysis, which is currently best known for leading to the development of Facebook, MySpace, and other Internet-based communities. Health care organizations such as our own are studying whether similar social networks might improve the effectiveness of interactions among large groups of clinicians in different locations, many of whom have not actually met each other before.

A generation ago, physicians either did not share the care of sick patients with other colleagues or relied mainly on other physicians who they saw in the hospital in the course of their workday. Today, clinicians are struggling to learn how to work with colleagues they rarely or never see—contributing to the chaos described in the first section of this book. A shared EMR is an important tool for helping them work together, but it seems likely that health care will need to learn lessons from social network humanware experts in the years to come.

The financial and cultural barriers to provider change are formidable, and the new skills that are needed to lead the change are difficult. But the goal of better organized, more reliable, and more efficient health care is compelling. In the next chapter, we turn to changes in the payer segment of the health care system that can help speed progress.

11   Payment Change

We have argued throughout this book that health care can improve as providers adopt systems that bring organization to care, and we believe that this evolution is under way. But this improvement will come too slowly if the only drivers are the desire of individual providers to give excellent care, and the gradual replacement of older physicians by younger clinicians who are more computer savvy and team oriented. Improvement can and should be accelerated by environmental forces, and in this chapter, we will examine the potential role of changes in the financing of health care.

Some of our fellow physicians may bristle at the notion that providers need external "nudging" to improve health care. But the fact is that providers *do* need help. Throughout most of the U.S. health care system, doctors work in small groups or solo physician practices, and most of these practices do not work closely with the hospitals to which they admit patients. Tightly structured systems that run hospitals and also employ the doctors who work in them are the exception, not the rule.

Neither collaboration nor the pursuit of efficiency are natural acts in a fee-for-service payment system in which doctors are paid for each individual patient encounter, and hospitals are paid for each day of hospitalizations or service provided. But this fragmented payment system and the fragmented state for providers have endured because of a chicken-egg problem. Without a change in the payment system, providers have little incentive to become more organized, and unorganized providers have difficulty accepting payment under any structure other than fee for service. Helping preserve the status quo is the appropriate reluctance of national health insurance companies that are serving national employers to implement different payment models for different provider groups in different regions. Such complexity raises the risk of major mistakes, and so the safer short-term course for these health insurance companies is to pay providers on a fee-for-service basis and try to hold the payments as low as possible.

One more factor that impedes provider organization, at least in some marketplaces, is ambivalence on the part of employers and insurance companies about providers coming together in any larger organization. On the one hand, purchasers want providers to work together more efficiently; on the other, purchasers fear that organized groups of providers will negotiate for higher payments.

In this chapter, we will discuss this purchaser ambivalence toward provider organization, and how it could and should evolve. We will then explore the major options for paying for health care, which have been introduced in chapters 8 and 9. In these prior chapters, we described how these payment models work, and some of their strengths and risks. We will focus here on their ability to drive change among providers. Before moving on to other market drivers of changes in the next chapter, we will also look at three forms of payment dysfunction that should be addressed in the course of efforts to achieve payment reform: administrative complexity, underpayment by government payers, and cost shifting to consumers.

Purchaser Ambivalence toward Provider Organization

Health insurance companies appreciate the potential of provider organizations to improve care, but their perspectives are complex. Not surprisingly, the reasons are financial. Fragmented providers (e.g., isolated one or two physician practices) must generally accept whatever fees are offered by an insurance plan or decide that they will not see patients covered by that plan. If an insurance company has more than a few patients in an individual doctor's practice, physicians usually knuckle under and accept whatever the insurance company is offering rather than risk losing patients. For small physician practices with little administrative infrastructure, the financial case for even taking the time to try to open negotiations with the health insurance company is weak. It is simpler and easier to just accept the payment schedule that the insurance company offers, and then just work harder to achieve their income goals.

Hospitals do the same. These facilities have more administrative staff and a greater ability to engage in negotiations with insurance companies, but still often accept contracts that cover their "marginal costs" (i.e., the incremental costs of taking care of additional patients), even if they do not cover "fully loaded costs" (i.e., the total costs of running the institution divided by the number of patient admissions). Applied on any scale, this approach spells trouble for any institution, since the health plans that are paying fully loaded costs seek to drive their payment levels down to those who are paying less. But hospitals frequently need to focus on the short run simply to survive the year financially and cannot risk losing even a small percentage of their patients. So they agree to contracts that do not cover their full costs.

Thus, contract discussions between insurance plans and providers who are isolated or in small groups barely qualify for the term negotiation. In fact, insurance plans often just inform providers what they will be paid—the most prominent example being the biggest insurance plan of all, Medicare. The insurance plans are of course seeking to hold rates as low as possible, and therefore give out increases that they believe are *just* large enough to keep providers from leaving their network.

The contracting teams at insurance plans are not malevolent people, even if our provider colleagues sometimes characterize them as such. Our (admittedly rosy) assessment is that most people working in health care share idealistic values or they might seek a less neurotic business. The management teams of insurance plans, however, are appropriately focused on the competitiveness of their companies. That competitiveness requires that they sustain a large population of members, so that the overhead costs of the insurance plans can be distributed across as many paying customers as possible, thereby making their insurance products attractive from a price perspective. Greater market share also enables them to seek "discounts" from hospitals and physicians.

So it makes perfect sense that insurance plan contracting teams try to sign providers to contracts that pay *just* enough to keep them from leaving the plan's network, and worry about any organization of providers into a group that might threaten to leave the plan's network together unless it receives higher payments. The actual underlying costs that providers must face are not an immediate concern for these contracting teams. In truth, the U.S. health care marketplace is quite heterogeneous, and it is difficult to make valid generalizations about trends that apply to the entire country. Yet as shown in figure 11.1, there has been an ebb and flow to annual increases in U.S. health care premiums over the last two decades. These shifts reflect market forces at work, with consolidation first among employers and then among providers.

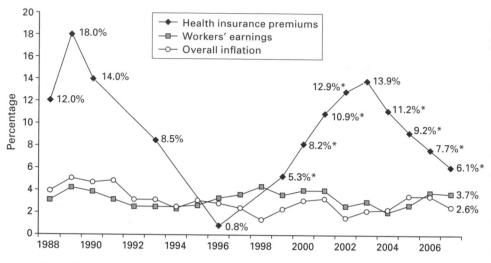

Figure 11.1
Average percentage increase in health insurance premiums compared to other indicators, 1988–2007. (Reproduced with permission of Employer Health Benefits 2007 Annual Survey, Henry J. Kaiser Family Foundation and HRET, September 2007, available at <http://www.kff.org/insurance/7672/sections/ehbs07-1-1.cfm>)

Under old-fashioned indemnity insurance in the early 1990s, physicians and hospitals had the upper hand in their relationships with health insurance plans. After all, patients then and now tended to be loyal to the people taking care of them, so providers could set prices that met their costs, even if those costs were well above consumer price inflation. In an effort to control these costs, employers aggregated their negotiating power through HMOs, which often had enough share of providers' patients to make "take it or leave it" offers to hospitals and physicians. The mid-1990s were thus the "good old days" to employers and insurance plans—when health care inflation was considered tamed.

The true underlying costs of health care continued to go up throughout this period, of course. New drugs (e.g., statins for cholesterol control) reached the market. New radiology technologies like functional MRI became common. Operating rooms were remodeled to accommodate new technologies like laparoscopic gall bladder removal (cholecystectomy). A nursing shortage developed nationally, leading to higher salaries for nurses—who constitute 30 to 40 percent of costs for most hospitals.

The tension between the increase in costs of providing care and payments that did not keep pace forced hospitals and physician practices to tighten their belts, and then tighten them again. In truth, this tension led to much needed management discipline among health care providers; this is, after all, how market forces are *supposed* to work. The pressure for efficiency drove decreases in hospital length of stay that were considered impossible a decade before. These pressures also caused many hospitals to close, and led others to merge in an effort to hold down their costs. Physicians also began to come together in various organizational structures—which usually had the goal of negotiating better contracts with insurers.

Once excess capacity had been driven out of the market and providers started to form networks, prices could not be driven down further. Nevertheless, health insurance plans were not completely opposed to providers becoming organized in the 1990s. In some parts of the country, health insurance plans promoted capitation—that is, they gave providers a fixed budget per member, and the providers could make profits if actual expenses were lower. Providers could also lose money, if spending was higher. We explored some of the problems that plagued capitation in the 1990s in chapter 9, and will look at its ability to drive provider organization shortly, but the key point for the immediate discussion is that physicians needed to be in some kind of group in order to accept capitation. After all, accepting financial risk for health care costs on an individual physician basis is considered too risky from a statistical basis.

Because capitation seemed like the best way to get physicians intensely interested in efficiency, health plans encouraged providers to move from their fragmented state into some kind of organization that could take responsibility for a population of patients. Today, this need has reemerged in a call for the development of "accountable care organizations" or "accountable care systems" [1, 2], but the notion that providers should become organized was a new one in the 1990s. And the most urgent focus for the organization of providers at that time was enabling their assumption of financial responsibility for a population— even if these newly organized groups had limited experience or systems for management of their patients' care.

In marketplaces where health plans pushed capitation aggressively, providers had three main options. First, physicians could join some organized group that would accept the financial risk and responsibility of capitation. These organizations might be large physician groups or PHOs, comprised of a hospital (or hospitals) and the physicians who admit patients to it.

If physicians were not part of a group that could assume the financial risk, they could be part of the health plan's network of individual providers, often called an IPA. Physicians who were part of such an IPA would be paid fee for service, but some portion (e.g., 10 percent) would be withheld. If health care spending was about what had been budgeted, then those funds or a portion of them would be sent later to the doctor. If spending were higher, then the withheld dollars would be used to cover the deficit.

A key problem with the health plan IPA model is that individual physicians know that they have little, if any, influence on the overall amount of spending. They therefore tend to ignore the financial rewards that might result if they collectively practiced more efficiently or better coordinated their care. These individual physicians have to assume that they will not get the incentive funds. Thus, they just work harder to make up for the presumed 10 percent reduction in their fees—often generating more costs for the health plan as they do so.

The third and final option was that physicians could choose not to see patients from that health plan.

Many health plans favored first option, because a well-organized group of providers has at least a theoretical chance of organizing themselves in ways to improve efficiency and quality. But such provider organizations were a double-edged sword for health plans, since these organizations could also negotiate for higher payments—and even threaten to walk away from the negotiating table.

As figure 11.1 shows, health insurance premiums began to rise in the late 1990s. There were several reasons for this, including continued medical progress. During this period, though, provider organizations began demanding increased payments to cover their rising costs—not just during the previous year, but also to compensate for the period in the mid-1990s when providers had actually been absorbing the costs of medical progress.

Thus, premiums went up in the late 1990s in part because organized providers could negotiate more effectively than fragmented providers. In some markets, all but one hospital had closed; that remaining hospital had considerable negotiating power because if it refused to sign a contract with a health insurance plan, that insurer could not enroll members in that market. In other markets, health plans had encouraged the formation of PHOs and other hospital-physician organizations that could accept capitation-based contracts; now these organizations threatened to terminate contracts with health plans unless payments were increased.

As negotiations between payers and providers became more contentious in the late 1990s and early years of the next decade, health care purchasers and legal authorities began to question whether the organization of providers does more harm than good. The Federal Trade Commission and the Department of Justice held hearings in 2003, and published a report titled "A Dose of Competition," which warned that large provider organizations could negotiate higher payments as well as fight off competitive pressures for improvement in efficiency and quality [3].

The peaks and valleys in figure 11.1 in a sense reflect an economic war being fought with economic weapons. In the mid-1990s, health insurance plans shifted the burden of rising costs to providers. In the late 1990s, providers became organized enough to push back harder during negotiations, and premiums rose sharply. The rate of rise of insurance premiums began to fall again in about 2003 as health plans started sharing the impact of cost increases with patients, through tactics including reductions in benefits and increases in copayments and deductibles. As discussed in chapter 8, patients are not particularly happy about costs being shifted to them. The sawtooth pattern of figure 11.1 suggests that this most recent strategy will not work indefinitely, and that efforts to control costs will focus on providers again.

Having lived and worked through these times and issues, our assessment is that health care is best served by a relative balance of power between providers and payers, and hurt by an imbalance in either direction. If payers have all the negotiating power over fragmented providers, the result will be low prices but also little ability or motivation for providers to work together to improve care. If providers have all the negotiating power over fragmented payers, the result will be high prices, and the same lack of motivation to improve quality and efficiency.

If both payers and providers are relatively organized, negotiations can lead to contractual relationships that support the adoption of systems to improve care, including efficiency. Of course, if providers are unable to deliver on the promise of better care, then the market is better off with fragmented care at lower prices. Therefore, to justify arguments for a balanced relationship between payers and providers, the ultimate pressure is on providers to organize themselves in ways that improve care.

Our hope is that the trend line in figure 11.1 will not extend into the future as a sawtooth that reflects shifts in negotiating power between payers and providers. In the 1990s, providers assumed financial responsibility for populations of patients without much real organization and without the systems described in chapter 5. Many provider leaders understand the liabilities of the fee-for-service payment system, but they still have fresh memories of the problems of abrupt implementation of a payment system for which providers are not sufficiently organized.

The bottom line is that payers need providers to get organized. But providers need to show that they can, if organized, create value.

Payment Model Options

The options for paying providers range from fee for service to full capitation, with multiple intermediate models including pay for performance, case rates, and subcapitation [4]. Hybrids of these various options also are being used in some marketplaces, such as a blend of fee-for-service payments combined with a per member per month payment to support the medical home function described in chapter 7. As suggested by the figure shown in the introduction and chapter 9, providers' degree of organization influences the type of payment system with which they can work most comfortably and effectively.

These different payment models are increasingly seen not just as tools for containing costs and improving quality but also as levers for changing the organization of health care delivery itself. Experiments by individual health plans and Medicare are already under way throughout the country, as both providers and payers try to understand the requirements for success and the potential impact of these various models [4–7]. In the sections below, we will comment on the ability of some of the major models to drive provider organization and performance improvement.

Pay for Performance

Pay for performance is unlikely to be the road to salvation for the health care system, but it just might be the entrance ramp to that road. In pay for performance, providers are paid on a fee-for-service basis, but with some portion of the payment, either through a withholding or an additional incentive payment, contingent on quality- and efficiency-related performance targets. The number of such pay-for-performance experiments ongoing in the United States is increasing rapidly, and opinion leaders are urging even greater expansion, even though the impact of pay for performance on quality and efficiency is as yet uncertain [4, 7–15].

There is good reason for both skepticism and optimism about pay for performance. The skepticism reflects data on the actual impact on pay for performance to date, which have been tepid at best. Initially, payers focused pay-for-performance programs on correcting the underuse of beneficial services [10–12], such as screening tests for breast and cervical cancer as well as preventive measures for patients with diabetes.

Over time, however, the limitations of this approach have become clear [4, 12, 14, 15]. Providers tend to focus their improvement efforts on the specific targets, with surprisingly little improvement in spillover in other areas. The gains themselves have often been modest, and not surprisingly, actual cost savings have not resulted from incentives to correct underutilization. Furthermore, the provider organizations that have been most successful in obtaining pay-for-performance bonuses tend to be those that performed well *before* the incentive programs were in place. These groups tend to be better organized and more financially successful even before the bonus payments are taken into account, so pay for performance has been accused of helping the rich get richer.

Why, then, is there any optimism for pay for performance? One reason for advocating the expansion of pay for performance is that it is still a new and evolving approach to contracting, and tremendous variability characterizes the incentives and structure of the provider organizations that participate in pay-for-performance contracts. Thus, passing judgment on whether pay for performance can produce enough value to meet the marketplace's needs would be premature at this point.

Second, pay for performance can be seen as an initial incentive program that starts providers up the diagonal line of the figure shown in the introduction and chapter 9. In order to pursue meaningful pay-for-performance incentives, providers must become organized. Even physicians in small practices that seek incentive payments for modest quality goals (e.g., improving mammography rates) have to adopt systems to track their populations of patients. When the goals become more ambitious (e.g., actually improving the control of diabetes), those physicians must begin working in teams that educate and help follow those patients between office visits. When the goals begin to include efficiency targets (e.g., the number of hospital admissions), physicians and hospitals need to collaborate in their efforts to improve care.

Third, if pay for performance is seen as a change agent more than an end-state program for the health care system, it is more viable for the currently fragmented mainstream of U.S. medicine than the other payment models described below. These other models require intense collaboration among providers before they can even be contemplated. Thus, pay for performance is a reasonable first step for many providers.

Finally, concern that the relatively modest incentives that characterize most pay-for-performance programs will not be enough to motivate providers are likely to be proven wrong. Prospect theory, the developers of which won the Nobel Prize for Economics in 2002, argues that relatively small incentives attract disproportionate attention, particularly when framed as potential losses instead of bonuses [16]. In our own experience with pay for performance, we have been impressed that physicians and hospitals can be strongly motivated by the risk of losing small incentives. It frequently seems as if the annoyance of "leaving money on the table" is more important than the bonuses themselves.

The barriers to success through pay for performance for providers and the overall health care system are considerable. We believe that a critical determinant of the impact of pay for performance is the nature of the provider organization with which the contracts are negotiated, and that larger, better-organized delivery systems are likely to provide more value to the consumer under these arrangements. For example, physicians in small practices seeking to adopt EMRs face higher financial hurdles than physicians in large groups. Similarly, individual or small groups of physicians have a limited ability to reduce hospital admissions or influence the site of care to which patients are admitted (e.g., community versus tertiary institutions). Provider organizations that include community and tertiary hospitals as well as physicians can take such issues on, however.

These challenges are difficult even when health care providers are tightly integrated—but they are close to impossible when providers practice in small uncoordinated groups. Our early experience with pay for performance indicates that success requires a critical mass of both patients and providers. Physicians must organize themselves into groups with sufficient numbers of patients so that there is a reasonable likelihood that their performance will reflect their actual efforts, rather than chance alone. And there must be sufficient numbers of patients in pay-for-performance contracts so that investment in the systems required for success can be justified by financially stressed physicians and hospitals.

Case Rates and Bundled Payments

Pay for performance encourages but does not force providers to pursue improvements that go beyond having high personal standards for themselves. After all, providers can choose to ignore pay-for-performnce incentives, simply accept the underlying fee-for-service payments, and hope that they might get some of the rewards by luck. Case rates and bundled payments raise the stakes and demands for providers considerably, which is why there is so much interest in implementing this approach for Medicare [4–6] and other payers [17–20].

There are multiple versions of case rate and bundled payment methods, but they share the common theme of paying providers for an episode of care rather than for individual services. An episode might be a hospitalization, the period associated with an acute illness, or even for the care of a chronic disease for one year. Providers who are paid under these methodologies are rewarded if they figure out how to take good care of patients as efficiently as possible. And they can be punished if the patients end up needing more resources than the providers receive. Thus, providers are usually receptive only to case rate/bundled payment methodologies that pay for care they consider within their control.

The most familiar type of case rate is the diagnosis-related group (DRG) system under which Medicare and many commercial health plans pay for hospitalizations. Under DRGs, hospitals have an incentive to reduce the length of stay, and they have done just that over the last two decades. To accomplish this goal, hospitals have developed care coordination systems to help move patients as quickly as possible back to their home or an appropriate lower level of care.

A problem with the DRG system is that hospitals' incentives conflict with the financial interests of physicians who are being paid for each daily visit. Hospitals want to shorten the length of stay, while physicians actually make less money if the hospitals do so. This conflict has not caused too much tension because both hospitals and doctors want to help patients medically and keep them happy—interests that encourage both types of providers to want hospitalizations that are not too long but just long enough. Nevertheless, the difference in interests between hospitals and physicians is real, and one more factor that hinders collaboration between them.

This tension explains why the range of providers covered by hospitalization-related payments is likely to expand. Medicare and other payers are intensely interested in combining hospital and physician payments into a single bundle—that is, a single fee for the hospitalization to cover both the physician and the hospital costs [5, 6]. The logic is that providers who have to figure out how to divide the payment are more likely to be able to figure out how to collaborate to improve the care.

A second way in which the scope of payment is expanding is over time. Instead of paying just for hospitalizations, Medicare and other payers want to pay for episodes of care, so that providers have an incentive to do all they can to avoid additional hospitalizations or other costs. For example, as mentioned in chapter 6, the Geisinger coronary artery bypass graft program charges a single fee that covers hospital and physician payments not just for the surgery but also for any care related to complications during the next ninety days [17, 18]. Medicare is also seeking to put in place incentives that reward hospitals that are able to reduce readmissions—and punish hospitals with high rates of such hospitalizations. This type of payment system is leading hospitals to implement programs such as follow-up phone calls to check on whether patients are stable, understand their medication regimens, and have timely follow-up appointments with their physicians.

Episodes of care do not have to be based on a hospitalization. An episode could be an illness that requires only outpatient care (e.g., ear infection), or one that could be treated on an inpatient or outpatient basis (e.g., mild pneumonia). Or an episode could be defined as the care of a patient with a chronic disease over the course of a year. Organizations such as Prometheus Payment, Inc. are developing and testing models of payment for physicians in which they would receive a lump sum case rate for the care of such episodes [20].

The degree of organization of providers determines which models for case rates/bundled payments that they can consider. Hospitals that do not have close relationships with physicians have a difficult time with bundled payments. Effective teams are needed to achieve efficiencies within and beyond the walls of a hospital.

If the incentives to adopt case rates and bundled payments are strong, these payment methods could provide powerful motivation for physicians and hospitals to organize themselves so they can collaborate and improve their care. Hence, even if case rates and bundled payments only focus on a modest number of diagnoses, their influence may extend well beyond these patient populations.

Medical Home

The medical home (see chapter 7) is a philosophical concept more than a payment model, but this philosophy cannot be brought to life under a pure fee-for-service payment system. Therefore, the growing interest in the medical home is leading health plans to experiment with per member per month payments for physician practices that are ready to commit to providing coordinated, timely, patient-centered care. Most of these physicians are primary care, but some are specialist practices for patients with serious chronic diseases such as renal failure or cancer.

The most common type of payment arrangements for early experiments with medical home physician practices is a combination of fee for service with per member per month payments that are contingent on the practice meeting service and quality goals [21]. In some models, these practices can achieve additional bonuses for improved efficiency, such as might result from reduced admissions to the hospital. Medical home practices try to reduce admissions by checking on patients frequently during high-risk periods, such as right after a hospitalization or emergency department visit, via telephone or office visits.

On the one hand, the medical home does not require that physicians collaborate with hospitals. On the other hand, the medical home demands that physicians work with nonphysicians, such as nurses who stay in contact with patients in between office visits. These teams tend to work better when there are systems like EMRs that allow the clinicians to know what each other is doing. Because small physician practices may not have enough patients to make team care viable, the medical home approach may generate pressure on physicians to consolidate into larger practices—another important step down the road to organization.

Capitation

Capitation is more of a destination than a lever for provider change, and as we suggest in prior chapters, it may not be a destination that is attainable or sustainable for many provider organizations or patients. In the mid-1990s, capitation was expected to become a common, if not dominant, payment methodology, but by the turn of this century, provider groups were restructuring their contractual relationships to reduce the scope of their financial risk [21]. Many providers sustained major financial losses, and found capitation disruptive to their relationships with patients and colleagues. Today, these providers would be extremely reluctant to consider such contracts again.

But the fact is that capitation never died out completely, and it could well come back again. Capitation is still an important contracting model throughout the country for some tightly organized groups, and it remains particularly common in California. Capitation is also the model used for many physician groups that participate in Medicare Advantage products, the alternative to fee-for-service Medicare that covers about 20 percent of all Medicare beneficiaries. As cost pressures on health care intensify, health plans in many markets are raising the question of a return to capitation.

There is no question that capitation has greater potential to focus providers' attention on costs of care than any other payment system. Of course, the pressure to control costs can create conflicts with the imperative to deliver the best possible care for patients, but our experience suggests that providers are probably better positioned and better trained to deal with this tension than anyone else. So we think providers should not shun the idea of another try at capitation but instead try to figure out how to make it work better this time around.

The key ingredients for capitation's success are demanding that:

1. Providers should be well organized, in groups that ideally include hospitals, physicians, and other clinicians

2. The provider organization should have EMRs and other systems described in chapter 5 to help them coordinate their care

3. The patients should be strongly encouraged to keep their care within that provider organization so that the providers can coordinate the care

4. The capitated patient population should constitute a large enough proportion of the providers' care so that the providers are committed to the use of their care improvement systems

5. The budget should be negotiated so that it is adequate to give the providers a better than fifty-fifty chance—ideally, considerably better—of achieving a surplus, and the budget will therefore need to be adjusted for differences in the severity of illness and technological progress

6. "Stop-loss" insurance programs should be available to protect providers from devastating losses related to high cost patients

The concept of combining capitation as an incentive for efficiency and pay for performance to reward quality has been proposed in some markets. If progress is made on the six factors listed above, this hybrid model could be an attractive inducement to providers to organize and improve their care.

Payment Dysfunction: Three Key Issues

As health plans contemplate different payment models that might improve care by encouraging providers to organize their efforts, there are three key types of payment dysfunction that should be addressed. The first of these issues is administrative complexity. Both providers and health plans have legions of personnel whose roles are to struggle with the chaos associated with filing claims for payment under the fee-for-service system. Advocates for a single-payer system argue that the savings from administrative simplification could fund access to care for the uninsured in the United States. Even without the upheaval that a single-payer system would require, the multiple payers in the United States could collaborate and standardize their processes so that the administrative costs could be reduced. Optimism that multipayer systems can be compatible with lower health care costs is supported by data from northern European countries [22].

For provider organizations, the administrative costs may be exacerbated by the current trend to shift health care costs to patients (also known as consumers)—a second type of dysfunction that will be addressed in more detail in the next chapter. One reason is that providers often do not know just how much to collect from patients when their contribution is a deductible (i.e., some amount up to which the patient is responsible for all costs) rather than a fixed co-payment. For example, if a patient in a health plan with a deductible has already spent more than his or her total financial exposure, then the provider should not collect anything. A second reason is that providers are more likely to be saddled with costs associated with attempts to collect debts from patients who are unwilling or unable to pay their share of their health care costs. The net effect of these plans on providers is comparable to a modest fee cut—which means that costs must be shifted to other insurance products.

The third type of payment dysfunction is underpayment by government payers (Medicare and Medicaid) for their patient populations. These government payers are sensitive to the demands by voters to avoid new taxes, and because they do not need to negotiate with providers, they hold annual increases below consumer inflation. The result is that hospitals and physicians lose more and more on these populations each year, and have compensated by shifting the costs of care on to commercially insured populations—contributing to the double-digit increases in health insurance premiums experienced by many employers. This cost shifting threatens the viability of any type of payment reform effort by nongovernment payers.

As important as payment methods are for driving provider organization and improvement in care, provider financial incentives alone cannot shoulder the entire burden. Other market forces including public reporting and engaging patients' interest in efficiency and quality also have roles to play. These roles will be explored in the next chapter, which looks at needed market change.

12   Market Change

Any decent vision of a better health care system has the patient at the center. This book began with the description of the chaotic experience of one of our own patients, SC, an elderly woman with lymphoma and multiple other conditions, and more than ten doctors who do their best on her behalf, but sometimes give her conflicting messages and advice, or fail to answer her questions. Her care is actually more coordinated than that received by most patients, because most of her physicians are within a single organization and use the same EMR. But her physicians and she would agree that we collectively have plenty of room for improvement.

Smart and outspoken patients like her provide glimpses of the destination. In June 2008, as this chapter was being written, she joined three physicians (one of the authors, her pulmonologist, and her oncologist) in a group email over two days discussing recent findings from a CT scan of her chest. The patient and the three physicians all hit "Reply to All" as they planned the next steps. In July, she emailed all three to remind them of her preferences regarding end-of-life care.

The patient lives fifty miles away, and two of these three physicians have never actually met face-to-face. Getting them and the patient all together in the same place for just fifteen minutes would take weeks to arrange. But during that flurry of activity in June 2008, they had virtual group meetings every few days—an informal version of team care. We will never know if the patient's outcome was influenced by that coordination, but the patient at least had peace of mind that her principal physicians were working together and with her.

Does this type of coordinated care happen for every complex patient who receives care in our organization? We wish that were the case. We have spent much of our resources and energy over the last fifteen years creating the *potential* for such coordinated care—for example, getting all our physicians on the EMR, creating the ability for patients to communicate with us via secure email systems, and so on. Yet neither our doctors nor our patients are fully and effectively using these systems.

In this particular case, we have a highly intelligent and forceful person who is *demanding* that we do all we can to coordinate her care. She feels like her life depends on it. Her physicians sense her urgency and are responding. The focus of the previous chapter, the payment system, is simply not a factor that motivates her doctors to work together on her behalf. (She has traditional fee-for-service Medicare, and her physicians are not paid for anything other than procedures and face-to-face visits.)

In aggregate, patients like her constitute the market for health care providers. These patients may feel powerless as individuals, but they actually have the ultimate power in shaping the health care delivery system. If they become frustrated and angry with their care, they can move to other physicians and hospitals, and damage the reputations of providers that they have left.

Financially and psychologically, providers cannot survive if they disappoint too many of their patients. Doctors and hospitals might not even notice a 1 percent increase in their business, but those same providers have panic attacks if they see a 1 percent migration away from them. Even the threat of the loss of a small number of patients is enough to cause hospitals and physicians to pursue improvements that might minimize that risk.

SC is a model for the activated consumer who some believe will drive the transformation of health care. She appreciates the value of coordination of care, which is a major reason she drives fifty miles each way to see her physicians in Boston. She insists on making that long drive for some routine tests (e.g., bone density) because she wants the results to be in the information system used by her doctors.

But this activated consumer gets little help from publicly reported information on the performance of her doctors and hospitals. These data tend to define performance in terms of what physicians do as individuals—not how well they coordinate their efforts with the other doctors who are caring for the same patient. And rankings of hospitals based on any single condition (e.g., heart surgery mortality) do not really tell patients with multiple conditions which institution can best handle their complexity.

In this chapter, we examine the potential of market forces derived from patients' choices to drive organization and improvement in health care. We will consider two basic approaches aimed at moving patients to higher-quality and more efficient providers—thereby putting pressure on providers to improve their care. These two approaches are the public reporting of provider performance, and the introduction of insurance products in which patients have incentives to choose higher-performing physicians and hospitals. We will argue that both approaches have a role to play in the shaping of a better health care system, but also have significant limitations. And we will assert that these drivers of market change are most likely to be effective in the context of the multidimensional approach we describe in our next and final chapter.

Public Reporting

The public reporting of health care performance data has been spreading rapidly over the last decade, and is assuming new and interesting forms. In the 1990s, the initial focus was on health insurance plans, and the movement's leader was the NCQA. The NCQA's HEDIS measures were developed to drive competition among HMOs based on quality, because of concerns that HMOs would otherwise compete solely on price.

In the last decade, however, the spotlight has turned on providers. Hospital quality data are now reported by a wide range of organizations that are public (e.g., the U.S. Department of Health and Human Services' Web site, available at <http://www.hospitalcompare.hhs.gov>), private (e.g., <http://www.leapfroggroup.org>), and for-profit companies (e.g., <http://www.healthgrades.com>). Physician quality data were first reported for subsets of physicians, such as cardiac surgeons and cardiologists who performed balloon angioplasty, but are now widely available for primary care physicians and a growing number of specialties. More recently, public reporting on hospitals and physicians has begun to include data on patient satisfaction (also known as patient experience) and costs.

As public reporting has broadened in scope and detail, the debate about its impact has intensified. Its advocates contend that transparency is an essential ingredient to any vision of a better health care system. After all, financial incentives cannot be targeted through pay-for-performance contracts at every aspect of health care that needs improvement. Public reporting, in contrast, has the potential to exert pressure for improvement on providers on a wide range of issues.

Critics argue that public reporting can have negative consequences that are often overlooked. These unintended consequences include the misclassification of physicians or hospitals due to the reliance on data that fail to capture differences in the severity and complexity of illness. Critics also worry that physicians and hospitals might avoid sicker patients out of concern that these patients might drag down their statistics.

Despite these potential problems, advocates of public reporting respond that patients have a right to know the data, and that this information can help them find the best care and best value. Thus far, however, only a small percentage of patients appear to be looking at data on their insurance plans, hospitals, and doctors, and few are acting on them. Table 12.1 shows results from national telephone surveys by Harris Interactive in 2001 and 2005. In both years, the proportions of respondents who had examined these data were low, and the percentages that made changes were trivial. And there was no sign of a trend toward greater use as of 2005 [1].

More recent data from a poll of 1,007 Californians who were surveyed in late 2007 found that the percentage who had looked at a physician rating site increased to 22 percent, and the percentage who actually made a change in their physician based on these data was just 2 percent [2]. So a change in the patient use of these data may be occurring—but it is happening slowly.

Despite these findings, no one should assume that public reporting has no effects. There is little question that publicly reported data has

Table 12.1
Awareness and use of quality ratings among the general public*

Level of quality information reported	Survey year	Looked at quality information	Considered a change on the basis of ratings	Actually made a change
		Percent of general public		
Hospital	2001	22	4	2
	2005	21	4	2
Health plan	2001	18	4	<1
	2005	20	4	1
Physician	2001	13	2	<1
	2005	11	2	1

Note: *Data are from Harris Interactive, Strategic Health Perspectives, 2001–2005. (Reproduced with permission from [1])

an impact on providers, even if only a few of their patients are aware of the information. And numerous health plans and for-profit companies are trying to determine how to help consumers understand and become more interested in data on their care. No one believes they have solved this challenge as of yet, but providers would be foolish to assume that public reporting will fail to become more effective.

Public Reporting on Quality

There are a series of important questions to ask about publicly reported measures on quality, and the first is about their validity. Just how well do publicly reported measures correlate with how patients fare? The answer seems to be "somewhat, but not as much as one might hope."

Most publicly reported quality measures are based on research suggesting that more reliable performance should lead to better patient outcomes—but the harsh reality is that there are not many treatments that have as dramatic an impact on patients' survival as giving beta-blockers after a heart attack (see chapter 4). For most quality measures, the correlation between measured performance and patient outcomes is surprisingly weak. For example, one recent study examined the relationship between measures of quality of care for acute myocardial infarction, heart failure, and pneumonia at 3,657 U.S. acute care hospitals as reported on the Centers for Medicare and Medicaid Services Web site, Hospital Compare [3]. When the researchers compared the best quarter of hospitals with the worst quarter, the differences in death rates were 1 percentage point or less.

One interpretation of these data is that all U.S. hospitals may be delivering about the same level of care, good or bad. A second interpretation is that our current treatments have only a modest impact on these conditions, so that even when physicians give exactly the right treatments, the impact on survival is small. A third possibility is that existing measures do not capture the essence of excellent care.

One logical solution is to use more accurate information. Clinical data from medical records are richer in detail than administrative data, and are used in some states for analyses of specific, well-defined issues, such as mortality with cardiac surgery. These data are being publicly reported in New York and elsewhere on an individual physician basis. In these states, patients who are considering cardiac surgery can look up mortality rates for specific hospitals and individual physicians.

There is no argument that the use of actual clinical data from the medical record makes these cardiac surgical ratings more valid than quality ratings based on administrative data alone, but the expense of collecting these clinical data from medical records is considerable. And there are a limited number of conditions for which researchers know how to adjust for the impact of differences in the severity of illness. Even in the absence of such risk adjustment systems, mortality data for an increasing number of medical and surgical conditions are being reported on Web sites sponsored by state governments.

Despite the well-known methodological problems with data and the apparent lack of consumer interest to date, public reporting is a powerful stimulant for providers to launch quality improvement programs [4]. No hospital or physician can bear the notion of being below the median—even though half of them must be. As leaders of a provider organization, we see the impact of public reporting among our colleagues, who grumble about the data, but then turn to the issue of how we can get better.

But we also see public reporting produce misleading results and unintended consequences. For example, many community hospitals immediately transfer patients who are having major heart attacks to tertiary care centers that can perform procedures aimed at restoring blood flow to the heart of the stricken patient. This approach is exactly the right strategy for the patient, and can lead to relatively few deaths from heart attacks in that community hospital. The result, however, can also be public rankings of heart attack mortality data that suggest that the community hospital is the best place to go if one is having a heart attack, while the hospitals that accept the high-risk patients look worse.

At the two teaching hospitals in our organization, transfers from other institutions account for 12 to 13 percent of all admissions, but about 40 percent of the deaths. In theory, statistical analyses should be able to adjust for differences in the severity of illness of these and other sick patients, but no risk adjustment system is complete. For instance, the diagnosis of heart failure could mean a mild, moderate, or severe impairment of heart function—but analyses based on administrative data can only reflect whether heart failure was present at all. Clinical information (e.g., data on the function of the heart from the medical record) can improve adjustment for the severity of the illness, but there is no gold standard for how much risk adjustment is enough.

Even with the use of clinical information to adjust for the severity of the illness and the complexity of the patients, the fear remains that public rankings of performance might produce perverse effects. A cardiac surgeon, for example, might perform one hundred coronary artery bypass graft operations per year. The average mortality rate for this operation is about 2 percent, so that this surgeon might have just two bypass surgery patients die in the course of an entire year. Now imagine being that surgeon, and being asked to operate on a patient with severe heart damage after a heart attack. This patient might have a 50 percent chance of dying with surgery, but an 80 percent chance of dying without it. The patient would be better off if the surgeon operated—but the surgeon would have good reason not to do so.

When the right thing to do for a patient is obvious, physicians will virtually always do it—but there are broad gray zones in medicine in which the best strategy is not explicit. In those gray zones, it is often impossible to dissect the factors that influence physicians' decisions. Critics of public reporting worry that public rankings of individual physicians could influence decisions in ways that are not in patients' best interest. The risk of dragging down "performance" might inhibit physicians from attempting an audacious treatment strategy when audacity is exactly what a patient wants and needs. And some data suggest that cardiac surgeons in states with public reporting at an individual physician level *do* avoid sicker patients [5].

Our take is that public reporting has plenty of problems, but it does more good than harm. Proponents of the New York State approach to public reporting on cardiac surgery dispute studies indicating that surgeons are avoiding sicker patients, and note that surgeons in New York with the highest mortality rates have been more likely to stop performing surgery than colleagues with lower mortality rates [6]. Hospitals with poorer ratings are not really losing business, but these hospitals do seem to respond with the implementation of quality improvement programs. In short, patients may not be paying much attention to these programs, but the providers who are being profiled do.

Does public reporting actually change how patients fare? A comprehensive review published in 2008 concluded that public reporting *does* lead to quality improvement *activities* in hospitals—yet the impact on actual patient *outcomes* is not clear [7]. To be fair, changing patient outcomes (e.g., survival) is difficult, because the dominant determinant of outcomes is how sick patients are. To demand that public reporting on quality demonstrate improvements in patient outcomes is a high hurdle, and physicians perform tests and give treatments every day that have not passed this test. A reasonable summary of the state of the science is that we have not yet figured out completely how to use public reporting to drive improvement in quality [4, 8, 9], but the likelihood is that we will get better with time.

Public Reporting on Cost

If public reporting on quality is a potentially powerful force that can do more good than harm, it is not yet clear whether public reporting on cost does anything at all. In many marketplaces, the push for full transparency as well as giving the patient information on quality *and* cost is under way. In several states, information is being posted on state-sponsored Web sites on the amounts paid to hospitals for various procedures (e.g., total knee replacement or an outpatient CT scan of the head; see, e.g., <http://www.nhhealthcost.org>). Some insurers are also providing data on the prices of physicians and hospitals to their members (see, e.g., <http://www.myaetna.com> and <http://www .myuhc.com>). The theory is that such data will allow patients to function like consumers, and choose to get their care at places that have the best combination of quality and price. The backup theory is that even if patients do not move their business to less expensive providers, the publication of prices will exert pressure on providers who are paid more to hold their prices down.

Whether this approach to controlling costs will be effective is far from certain [10], and some experts believe that the public reporting of costs could actually *raise* health care spending. The reason for this counterintuitive effect is that patients tend to prioritize quality over price in health care, particularly when they are frightened or sick. An additional problem is that available measures of quality do not seem to capture well what patients value most, so patients do not believe that providers have similar quality even if publicly reported measures do not demonstrate a difference. Furthermore, if Hospital A costs more than Hospital B, patients might suspect that there *must* be a reason for the higher price—and they seek care at Hospital A. This "Neiman Marcus Effect" is exacerbated by the fact that most Americans are in insurance products that make them relatively insensitive to differences in the price of care. They are mainly concerned with their out-of-pocket costs, and are uninterested in or confused by information on the overall rates negotiated by insurance plans and providers.

If patients are not drawn to lower-priced providers, the reward for being lower priced does not exist. Therefore, a second way in which price transparency could raise costs is by "flattening" the market. When lower-priced providers learn what higher-priced providers are being paid, they tend to demand that the gap be closed. The Federal Trade Commission would never allow providers to share information on their contracted rates for just this reason.

Thus, the CBO gave a mixed review to the idea of price transparency in the "Economic and Budget Issue Brief" of June 5, 2008 [10]. Its key points are as follows:

- Most consumers are protected from the full price of health care, which limits their incentive to compare prices

- Physicians and other health care providers have the greatest influence over where patients receive care, because patients often do not believe they have the information needed to make such decisions

- An awareness of price has little impact on providers or patients in emergency situations, or in the small percentage of cases that account for most health care spending

- The publication of prices is likely to lead to a narrowing of the range of prices paid to providers, but such transparency could lead to increases rather than decreases in prices

If the CBO logic is borne out by regional experiments in price transparency, this strategy is not likely to be a powerful force for cost control, nor a catalyst for organization and the improvement of care. It might actually raise prices on a short-term basis. In the longer run, it could exert pressure on providers to hold down their prices, if a sufficient number of patients begin to move into insurance products in which they have significant exposure to the costs of care.

Excessive exposure to costs is, of course, just what insurance is intended to protect patients from. But some exposure would engage patients in the search for more efficient care. And that is the idea behind new insurance products in which patients share more of the costs of their care—the focus of the next part of this chapter.

Insurance Product Design

"Skin in the game": this unpleasant expression describes efforts to control health care expenditures by making patients more concerned about the costs of their care. The problem is that patients and providers are the main determinants of what happens in health care, but neither of these parties has much incentive to make sure resources are used as efficiently as possible. As long as someone else is paying the bill, patients and physicians are focused mainly on relieving patients' symptoms and fears as *quickly* and *effectively* as possible. Doctors and patients currently care about a different type of efficiency—one that places value on time and angst, not the insurer's dollars.

The idea of giving patients skin in the game means creating a context in which they might pause before going to a higher-cost doctor or hospital, because it will cost them more than if they seek care from a more efficient provider. In theory, the loss of even a modest number of price-sensitive patients would encourage providers to become more efficient so they could compete on price. Alternatively, providers could work harder to demonstrate that they offer superior quality—better patient outcomes, better service, and greater safety. Or providers could try to become more efficient in the overall utilization of resources—for instance, by reducing the use of high-cost radiology tests or lowering the rate of readmission of patients after hospitalization. If patients who sought care from them had a lower utilization of high-cost services, these providers could argue that they *deserved* higher prices.

In an ideal market, providers would try to do both: work relentlessly to become more efficient *and* improve their quality. In fact, leaders of organizations like Virginia Mason Medical Center maintain that efficiency and quality are two sides of the same coin, and that they require the same basic strategies. We agree, and think that the concepts of provider organization and system adoption that we have described in this book are in fact helping health care become better and more efficient—and that consumer pressure does spur their adoption.

But there are some flies in the ointment. The problems begin with the concept of shifting costs to patients, which conflicts with cultural expectations of what it means to be sick in most societies. These expectations are articulated most famously by Harvard sociologist Talcott Parsons as the sick role, which describes the social rights and obligations of the person with an illness [11]. The four key aspects of the sick role are that the patient:

1. Is exempt from normal social roles

2. Is not responsible for his or her condition

3. Should try to get well

4. Should seek technically competent help, and cooperate with the medical professional

The sick role works well for acute illnesses like pneumonia or a broken leg, and not as well for chronic illnesses or conditions that may result from lifestyle choices. After all, if someone has a chronic condition like diabetes, can that person be exempt from normal social roles forever?

Still, the idea of shifting costs to patients and requiring them to become savvy consumers at a time of illness conflicts with the notion that the sick person is exempt from normal social roles. Patients and their families tend to be focused on their illnesses and do not want financial considerations to be their responsibility. The result: enrollment in plans with major shifting of costs to patients has been low, and the people enrolled in them tend to be less happy about them [12].

A tough but logical response from those paying for health care (employers and government) might be: "We just can't afford your cultural expectations. We have tried everything else. When insurance companies tried to manage care, patients and doctors rebelled. We have not been successful in getting providers to control costs by changing the way we pay them. We don't have other options. We need you patients to care about costs, and the only way to do that is to put some of your skin in the game."

This response began to transition from rhetoric to reality in 2004, when Congress passed legislation establishing health savings accounts (HSAs), which were coupled with high-deductible health insurance plans (HDHP). These HSA-eligible HDHPs have lower premiums than traditional health plans, because the first expenses are paid for by the patient, not the health plan. Since most people do not spend more than $1,000 in health care costs in any given year, these insurance plans frequently pay nothing at all for the care of most of their members and only kick in when patients have major expenses.

Depending on one's perspective, these plans provide poor insurance or are exactly what insurance was intended to be. As is so often the case in health care, the fairest assessment is somewhere in between. Thus far, however, there are troubling concerns about *who* is signing up for these HDHPs and *why*.

In these plans, patients (or their family or employers) can deposit money into an HSA, which can be invested in the stock market like other retirement-oriented plans. These funds can be withdrawn as needed to pay for health care costs at any time—now, next year, or years after that. The theory is that the combination of lower premiums and the tax-free savings potential of HSAs should encourage people to sign up for health plans in which the first few thousand dollars of expenses are purchased with their own funds and that they will become savvier consumers, looking for the best value for their dollar.

The concern of skeptics of HSAs and HDHPs, however, is that they attract the wealthy and healthy. From the perspective of a financial planner, the ideal candidate for an HSA is someone wealthy enough to put money into an account and healthy enough that they would not need to spend that money on health care expenses. Contributions into HSAs up to the annual deductible of the HDHP are exempt from income tax, and withdrawals for medical expenses are not federally taxed. Contributions beyond the annual limit *are* taxed, and withdrawals for nonqualified expenses are also subject to taxes, and if withdrawn before age sixty-five, an additional tax penalty.

If the "investor" in an HSA does need to spend money on health care, he or she is best off if they pay for it out of other resources, rather than withdraw it from their HSA. Their financial return is maximized if they leave their money in the HSA untouched, so that it can earn profits, and then the profits can be earned on those profits—all free of taxes. Indeed, there are no more effective ways to shelter money from taxes under U.S. income tax policies than HSAs.

But our focus here is health care, not retirement planning, and HSAs are not expected to bring much financial value to those who are less wealthy or sick. Those less fortunate people might put money into an HSA, but then have to withdraw it immediately to pay for their care because they do not have other resources available to them. People with significant medical conditions often do not feel that they have the option to shop around for the best bargain; they are mainly focused on getting the best possible care for their illnesses. Thus, HDHPs and HSAs might attract the healthy and wealthy, leaving the sick and poor behind in traditional health plans, thereby causing the insurance premiums for those products to spiral upward.

Data demonstrate that these HSAs are being used more as tax shelters by the relatively wealthy than as tactics for savvy consumers of health care. An April 2008 report from the Government Accounting Office found that the average annual income of HSA enrollees was about $139,000, compared with $57,000 for those without HSAs [10]. In 2005, the total value of all HSA contributions was $754 million, but withdrawals were just $366 million. The greater the income of people who opened an HSA, the greater the gap between what they deposited and what they withdrew; in other words, the more people earned, the more they saved for the future in HSAs. Perhaps these unspent dollars will be spent for health care costs in later years, but these mismatches strongly suggest that HSAs are being used more to avoid taxes than support consumerism by patients.

The report found that the number of individuals covered by HSA-eligible plans increased from about 438,000 in September 2004 to about 4.5 million in January 2007. The number of tax filers reporting HSA activity also increased, but more than 40 percent of enrollees in HSA-eligible plans did not open an HSA. Presumably, these are people who sign up for a HDHP because of the lower monthly insurance premium, but do not have an employer or their own resources to deposit money into an HSA. More than a third of surveyed employers that offered HSA-eligible plans made no HSA contributions on behalf of their employees. These HDHP enrollees without HSAs are making the gamble that they will remain healthy and not have to pay higher insurance premiums that would be used to subsidize the care of those who become sick.

Do HDHPs help or hurt health care? The data are unclear [14]. There is no question that patients with high deductibles use fewer resources, and there are some encouraging signs that these patients tend to filter out some lower-value services. For example, one recent study found that people with traditional health insurance who switched to an HDHP visited the emergency department less frequently, and that the reductions seemed to be mainly in repeat visits for conditions that were of relatively low severity [15].

Another recent study compared the use of preventive care before and after the introduction of an HDHP in a Massachusetts HMO [16]. This HDHP fully covered Papanicolaou tests, mammography, and fecal occult blood testing to screen patients for cervical, breast, and colon cancer, but did not provide full coverage for colonoscopy, flexible sigmoidoscopy, or barium enemas for routine screening. The HMO found that enrollees who switched into the HDHP had the same rates of cancer screening as before, but they did have a 27 percent drop in the use of colonoscopy, flexible sigmoidoscopy, and barium enemas. In short, these members seem to have substituted a less expensive test that was fully covered by their health plan (fecal occult blood testing) for the more expensive tests that were no longer fully covered. The incentives worked.

Decades of health services research, though, suggests that when patients have to bear a greater proportion of the costs of their care, they *do* use fewer resources, but their choices are far from perfect. They skip tests that they should undergo and fail to fill prescriptions that they need. For example, a recent study examined what happened with employees of one large manufacturer that offered HDHPs in 2004 alongside of traditional insurance options [17]. Compared with enrollees in traditional plans, employees who chose an HDHP had fewer medical problems and lower baseline pharmaceutical costs. They were also more likely to be managers in the company than "line" employees—for instance, 33 percent of those in the HDHP were paid by the hour versus 85 percent of those with traditional insurance.

Despite their greater average income, 17 percent of the patients in HDHPs stopped taking their medications for hypertension over the next year versus 5 to 6 percent of those with lower-cost exposure. Similarly 17 percent stopped taking their cholesterol medications, compared with 6 to 7 percent of those with lower-cost exposure. The use of generic medications *was* statistically higher among employees in HDHPs, suggesting that the financial incentives were doing some good as well as some harm. But if the true bottom line of health care is addressing medical issues, national survey data suggest that people with a wide variety of conditions are more likely to forgo filling a prescription if they are enrolled in an HDHP (table 12.2) [1].

Skepticism also remains about the direct potential cost-savings impact of HDHPs. Many employers are encouraging enrollment in HDHPs by offering significant contributions into employees' HSAs—and after the premium and the HSA contribution are added up, costs are similar to or even higher than what the employer might have paid as an HMO premium. The employers are pursuing this strategy because they believe the longer-term rate of rise of costs for people with skin in the game will be lower.

A more important limitation for the cost-saving potential of HDHPs is that a small number of people (only about 3 to 5 percent of patients) account for half of health care spending. There is only so much cost sharing that these people can bear, and one might safely assume that most of these unfortunate families are already under financial duress.

As time goes by, the insurance plans are getting more sophisticated, and efforts are being made to minimize the risk of perverse incentives. For example, some employers and health plans are avoiding patient

Table 12.2
Proportion of members of high-deductible health plans and other privately insured patients who did not fill a prescription because of cost*

Condition for which medication was prescribed	Patients enrolled in non-high-deductible plan	Patients enrolled in high-deductible plan
	Percent	
All	13	28
Diabetes	15	24
Depression	9	30
Arthritis	9	16
Chronic pain	9	23
Heart disease or hypertension	8	18
Allergies	7	23
Asthma	9	23
High cholesterol	2	16
Other chronic condition	17	25

Note: *Data regarding patients in non-high-deductible plans are from a random digit-dial telephone survey of adults in private health plans who report that their deductibles are less than $1,000 for single coverage and less than $2,000 for family coverage. Data for patients in high-deductible plans are from an online survey of adults in private health plans who report that their deductibles are $1,000 or more for single coverage or $2,000 or more for family coverage. A total of 438 patients enrolled in a non-high-deductible plan and 916 patients enrolled in a high-deductible plan were surveyed, and the given conditions were reported by the following numbers of patients in each group: diabetes, 31 and 71, respectively; depression, 69 and 196; arthritis, 85 and 229; chronic pain, 60 and 156; heart disease or hypertension, 129 and 295; allergies, 140 and 374; asthma, 51 and 135; high cholesterol, 131 and 274; and other chronic condition, 96 and 234. The percentages were calculated on the basis of weighted figures. All data are from Harris Interactive, Strategic Health Perspectives, 2005. (Reproduced with permission from [1])

cost exposure for the care of chronic diseases like diabetes or hypertension; it is in no one's interest, after all, to have patients skip doses of their medications and develop preventable complications of such diseases. Aetna has reported data showing that 17,411 people who were continuously enrolled in an HDHP that completely covered preventive and screening services did not reduce their use of such care at all [18].

In this "value-based purchasing" approach, patients *are* exposed to costs for acute problems like getting a CT scan for headaches. But health insurance plans have also realized that exposing patients to a share of the costs for hospitalizations does not provide much financial incentive for shopping, since patients tend to exceed their maximum exposure quickly. The plans are instead focusing their cost-sharing efforts on outpatient care, like radiology and pharmaceutical treatments, where patients might pause before allowing resources to be expended.

Enrollment in HDHPs remains low, in large part because patients and providers just do not like them. Patients do not want to have to think about costs when they are sick, and providers do not like having their performance measured by insurance companies trying to help their members act more like consumers. In addition, providers have a difficult time collecting payments from patients responsible for the first $1,000 or $2,000 of their care, so these HDHPs actually lead to lower revenue.

Nevertheless, a survey in 2008 showed that large employers and health plans have made progress in putting in place the building blocks for a consumer-oriented vision of the health care marketplace [19], and many experts believe that HDHPs will ultimately account for 10 percent or more of the commercial insurance marketplace. Tax policies affecting HDHPs may be refined to encourage employers and employees to contribute more into HSAs.

Furthermore, efforts to achieve universal health care coverage for Americans may well adopt the "individual mandate" approach used in Massachusetts, in which healthy people pay a hefty fine if they do not buy health care insurance. In the absence of an individual mandate, the gamble logically taken by many healthy people is to go without coverage. In the presence of an individual mandate, the gamble is to buy insurance with a high deductible rather than more costly insurance products with lower exposure to costs. If these healthy individuals buy HDHPs, they are at least contributing some funds into the pool needed to pay for care for those who are or become sick.

A variant on the skin in the game theme that will probably have a smaller market penetration is the tiering of providers, so that patients pay higher co-payments if they choose to go to more expensive or lower-quality hospitals and doctors. This tiering approach annoys providers because of inevitable problems in the methods used to assess their quality—particularly those who get less than stellar evaluations. Physician groups in some states have filed or threatened legal action challenging the methods used to assign physicians to tiers. Yet an argument for the tiering approach is that it puts less pressure on the patient to be a consumer than do HDHPs. Patients who sign up for tiered products have to make some judgment about *where* they choose to receive their care, but are not pressured to make financially based decisions about *whether* they undergo various tests and treatments.

HDHPs may upset patients, and tiered insurance products may upset providers, but their influence on the overall health care system is undeniable. These influences include:

• A focus on the patient as a consumer. While providers remain ambivalent about the blurring of these two roles, there has been a definite increase in the pressure on providers to improve patients' experience of care and find ways to meet patients' needs outside of doctor-patient visits such as electronic interfaces with their medical records.

• Health plans, even conventional ones, have given new emphasis to putting tools in the hands of patients to follow their health issues. There is anecdotal evidence that patients who sign up for HDHPs tend to be more active participants in their own care (e.g., using Web sites or getting more preventive exams). Whether they were more active before enrolling in these plans is not known.

• Provider organizations (including ours) are taking the initiative and publishing information on their quality and efficiency on the Internet and paper. The provider logic is that as long as information is going to be published, they should have a role in shaping the story. Whether consumers are looking at this information is unclear, but the publication of these data puts pressure on providers to improve their care—a pressure that we consider healthy.

A *balanced* assessment at this point is that insurance products that give patients skin in the game probably do both good and harm, and no one knows exactly which way the scales will tip in the long run. That assessment might argue for caution in spreading these models of insurance. After all, a basic principle of medicine is primum non nocere ("first do no harm"), and if an HDHP were a new drug, it is unlikely that the FDA would approve it.

A *realistic* assessment is that HDHPs and other insurance products that put patients' skin in the game are here to stay, because the cost pressures in health care are so intense. The financial downturn of 2008 is intensifying the challenge for employers to provide *any* health insurance coverage at all for their employees, and HDHPs are better for patients and providers than higher rates of uninsured Americans. Thus, the goal for providers, patients, and purchasers of care should be to work collaboratively with health plans to refine the models, so that the ratio of benefit to harm continues to improve.

An *optimistic* assessment is that HDHPs and public reporting are part of an environment that is encouraging innovation in care. There seems little question that health care in the future will give patients much more information—clinical, price, quality, and other types of data. Much remains unknown about what information is most useful and how it should be presented. But information for patients will surely be a critical part of an overall strategy for improving health care—the focus of our final chapter.

13 Accelerating Evolution

The central argument of this book is that the organization of providers is an essential step in the development of a better health care system. Organization enables providers to bring order to the chaos generated by technological progress. Organized providers can use EMRs, patient registries, disease management programs, and other systems described in this book to make health care more efficient, reliable, and safe.

Perhaps because we are optimists, we believe that the adoption of such systems and the resulting improvement in health care is already under way. But because we are realists, we know that the pace of improvement is not fast enough. Rising costs threaten access to care for tens of millions of Americans—which is reason enough to confront the barriers that slow the evolution of health care.

In our prescription for improving health care, we assign the greatest responsibility to our own colleagues—the providers of health care. This provider-focused perspective is shared by nonproviders who assert the need for a "market-based but physician-led" future for health care [1]. Physicians and other clinicians could surrender to their fear of uncertainty and try to delay inevitable change. Or they can play their more appropriate leadership role and actively shape the development of a better health care system.

There are good reasons why many health care providers have not embraced this role with enthusiasm to date. The financial stakes for providers are high, and their current profit margins are thin. Many organizations do not have the financial reserves or access to capital for major investments in information technology and other structural needs.

The cultural issues are even more formidable. Organized care requires physicians to surrender some of their individual autonomy and work in teams. They must learn new computer and interpersonal skills, and adjust to new types of incentives.

Providers need help in addressing these issues. As we will discuss, health insurance plans, employers, patients, and health policymakers all have roles to play in facilitating change. But the ability of health care providers to rise to the occasion will dictate how quickly high-performing health care systems develop in the United States. Collectively, we need to create an environment that makes it possible for providers to lead the change—and unwise for them not to.

Multiple Strategies

A first step in the development of a better health care system is acceptance that no *single* solution to our problems exists. No single payment system such as capitation or a single market strategy such as consumer activation can drive the needed change. Every potential strategy offers some potential benefits, but each one also has potential liabilities. To advocate any single strategy is to invite skepticism and consolidate resistance to that approach.

A more productive approach is to accept that we have to pursue *several* strategies simultaneously. Every one of those strategies will have its flaws; after all, whenever money changes hands, there is the potential for perverse consequences. Each strategy should be used in ways that maximize the benefits and minimize the risks. Through the thoughtful management of financial and nonfinancial incentives, we believe the pace of improvement in health care can be accelerated.

For providers, a difficult challenge is the transition from critic to playwright. Providers should continue to speak out about what they oppose, but they also have an obligation to say what they are for. If we providers are to be serious participants in shaping the health care marketplace, we actually have to be supportive of *several* strategies for improving efficiency and quality—even though each and every one will generate angst among our colleagues. Our job as provider leaders is not to fight change but rather to mitigate risk and optimize effectiveness as multiple strategies are deployed.

So what potential strategies exist, and what are their likely effects? We have our own opinions, of course, but to get broader input, we conducted an informal survey of twenty-six health care leaders from the United States and the United Kingdom who were attending a meeting in Boston in July 2008. These experts included government officials, economists, health plan executives, and provider leaders. We

Table 13.1
Ratings of potential impact of various strategies on quality and efficiency

Strategy	Quality (0 to 5)	Efficiency (0 to 5)
Public reporting	3.4	1.5
Pay for performance with fee-for-service payment system	2.9	2.5
Medical home supported by both fee for service and per member per month payments	3.1	2.9
Case rates and bundled payments for physicians and hospitals	2.8	3.2
Capitation for organized delivery systems	3.2	4.0

Note: 0 = no beneficial impact; 5 = high potential impact

asked them to rate each of five strategies on their potential effectiveness for driving improvement in quality and efficiency. A rating of 0 would indicate no beneficial impact at all, while a rating of 5 meant a belief in major potential impact. The average ratings are shown in table 13.1. (Note that the authors did not vote.)

As shown in table 13.1, the twenty-six policy experts thought that public reporting had the greatest potential for improving the quality of care and the least impact on efficiency. In a discussion of their ratings, these experts said that public reporting could include data for literally hundreds of performance measures. Even if only a few patients took note of these data, the data put healthy pressure on providers to improve in areas for which they are below average.

On the other hand, virtually all of these experts were skeptical that the public reporting of cost data would moderate cost trends. As noted in chapter 12, these experts felt that consumers would not be interested in cost information unless they were responsible for a large proportion of the costs of care, but large increases in patients' cost exposure could be harmful to poorer patients and were not likely to be politically acceptable. If anything, patients might be drawn to higher-cost providers because of suspicion that the care might be better in ways that were not captured by available quality measures. The publication of cost data also can be expected to encourage lower-paid providers to seek increases to match rates of better-paid competitors.

Pay-for-performance contracts that consist of bonuses for improvement in addition to fee-for-service payments were expected to have modest impacts on quality and efficiency. The consensus was that pay for performance leads to intense attention on the specific measures that are the focus of the incentives, but that spillover improvement effects in other areas are disappointingly small. In other words, if providers have an incentive to improve diabetes care, they will do so, yet there is no particular reason to expect improvement in care for other conditions. Financial incentives can only be offered for a small number of quality goals, while public reporting can exert pressure on providers across a broad spectrum.

Pay for performance has the ability to improve efficiency on some targeted areas, such as increasing the use of generic medications. This group of experts, however, thought that bonuses for efficiency cannot overcome the "undertow" of fee for service's incentive to deliver more care. That said, pay for performance under fee for service helps get physicians organized, and that can be an important step toward the use of some strategies with greater potential for enhancing efficiency.

The medical home approach represents a hybrid model of payment for physicians (usually primary care physicians, but also including specialists who might assume the major responsibility for caring for patients with conditions such as cancer or kidney failure). In many medical home models, physicians are paid a fee for service for each individual office visit, so they are rewarded for extra efforts to see patients when visits are needed. On the other hand, the physicians are also paid monthly fees (per member per month), so that they receive a financial reward if they can meet their patients' needs in other ways. If physicians do not provide good care and good service, they are at risk for losing both types of payment. But if they provide excellent care and are creative in meeting their patients' needs, they can potentially have a greater income than they would with pure fee-for-service payments.

The medical home is a relatively new concept and actually exists only in pilot projects around the United States. Nevertheless, enthusiasm for its potential impact among these experts was reflected in moderately high scores for both efficiency and quality, even though the medical home's incentive payments are focused only on just one doctor per patient. The hope is that this doctor will find ways to improve quality and lower costs by doing things like scheduling patients' visits shortly after hospital discharge to be sure that they are taking the right medications.

Case rates and bundled payments, such as the Geisinger approach to coronary artery bypass surgery described in chapter 6, had similar scores to the medical home. When this approach is applied to hospital-based care, it requires physicians and the hospital to work together to optimize efficiency and quality of care. If they cannot figure out how to collaborate, they are collectively at risk for losing money or patients. The impact of this approach is limited somewhat by the modest number of procedures and types of patients for which case rates can be easily applied.

Capitation for an organized delivery system had the highest expected impact on efficiency (4.0), since this group of experts believed that well-organized providers can manage resources more effectively than any other available option. What was surprising was that these experts also had high expectations for the quality of care under capitation. The reason that they gave during a discussion of their ratings was that capitation required providers to become highly organized, and that organization could make possible major gains in quality as well as efficiency.

These ratings are only the opinions of a modest number of experts at one meeting. Not every possible strategy for improving efficiency and quality was evaluated, and there are certainly other options that could have been considered, including hybrids of these models. Still, these ratings imply that public reporting is an important tool for improving quality—but not useful for containing costs. Various payment systems offer the potential to improve both quality and efficiency, but as we suggested in chapter 9, payment systems should be matched to the degree of provider organization. There is no one size that fits all.

In sum, optimal performance should be sought by invoking multiple strategies including public reporting to drive quality, and the development of a flexible payment system approach that encourages the organization of providers as well as rewards both quality and efficiency.

Confronting Myths

To use multiple strategies simultaneously, health care's stakeholders must have a common understanding of the strengths and weaknesses of the various approaches. That requires confrontation of some common myths, so that time and effort are not expended on false hopes. Opinions differ among various experts, but the following are our perspectives on five widely held but flawed beliefs.

Choice Equals Quality

U.S. patients treasure the freedom to go to any physician or hospital they choose, and resent any effort to restrict their options. They cannot judge the quality of providers from the data available to them, so they rely on the recommendations of doctors, family, and friends. They suspect that health plans or provider organizations that try to keep their care within some subset of providers are doing so for financial reasons, and these suspicions are often correct.

The irony is that the freedom to go to any provider leads to the fragmentation of care, and that fragmentation worsens quality. As this chapter was being written, SC, the patient described in chapter 1, was admitted emergently to a hospital in Rhode Island for pneumonia. Multiple tests including a CT scan of her chest and a bronchoscopy (in which a tube is inserted into the lungs) were repeated by physicians who did not seem to know that these tests had been performed in Boston in recent months. Her doctors there also gave her medicines for a presumed diagnosis of heart failure. They did not know that her heart function had been normal on recent tests performed in Boston and at another hospital in Rhode Island.

In this case, the patient had no choice except to go to the nearest hospital at the time she was stricken, but many patients voluntarily fragment their care. They may end up with a cardiologist at one hospital, a gastroenterologist at another, a primary care physician at a third, and no reliable form of communication among these doctors. The care of such patients would be better if they valued integration among their physicians more than the freedom to go anywhere.

Confronting this myth is difficult, because U.S. patients *want* to be able to go wherever they choose. They value choice almost above affordability of care, so only marked decreases in their costs cause patients to give up the freedom to go where they want. They seem to value choice above value itself. They do not realize that average physicians who work closely together might help them more than brilliant physicians who do not.

Trying to persuade consumers to give up choice is unlikely to be a successful strategy. Health insurance products, however, can provide incentives for patients to keep their care within an organized group of providers, and organized groups of providers can create and use systems that truly make it more valuable for patients to remain within their organization. The more that patients are willing to keep their care within an organized provider network, the more feasible it is for those providers to accept prospective payment systems such as capitation.

Higher Quality Will Reduce Costs

We really wish this myth were true. Unfortunately, it is not—at least not completely. There are some "sweet spot" issues for which better quality really does reduce costs. For example, programs that reduce complications for hospitalized patients and decrease their rates of readmission to the hospital often do save money while improving patients' outcomes. But the harsh reality is that better quality generally means higher costs, not lower ones.

We emphasize this unpleasant truth because politicians campaigning for office frequently say that they will reduce health care costs through better preventive care. Note, though, that once they are elected, they do not try to fund health care through savings from prevention. The reason is that those savings never materialize. Prevention requires medications and patient education, both of which are costly. And sooner or later, everyone does become sick and expire—generating considerable health care costs in the process.

This issue was analyzed recently by experts from the American Diabetes Association, American Heart Association, and American Cancer Society [2]. Using data on a national sample of people, they concluded that about 78 percent of adults age twenty to eighty alive today are candidates for at least one prevention intervention. If every single person received those interventions, heart attacks and strokes would be reduced by 63 and 31 percent, respectively. Yet these health benefits would be achieved at a price. The only preventive activity that is actually likely to be cost saving over thirty years is smoking cessation. Other preventive interventions such as the control of blood pressure, diabetes, and cholesterol would substantially increase overall health care costs.

When preventive care is focused on patients with a high risk for hospital admissions, such as patients with known heart disease, cost savings from avoided hospitalizations might actually offset the expense of the preventive care. But when preventive programs are focused on lower-risk or completely healthy patients, they often do not save money. Some preventive programs actually require more to "buy" a year of life than liver transplantation programs [3].

A major movement is afoot to withhold payments to hospitals when patients suffer serious reportable events (also known as "never events") such as surgery on the wrong site or the wrong patient, or operations in which a foreign body (e.g., a clamp or gauze pad) is left behind in the patient. These events are horrifying when they occur, of course, but the financial savings from withholding payment for these events will be minimal. The events are rare, and many hospitals do not seek payment when such events have occurred.

In our own organization, we invest heavily in information systems and other initiatives to improve quality and safety. We look carefully at the financial implications of these initiatives. For most of these investments, the return on investment is care that is better, but not cheaper.

That said, we believe that there are opportunities to reduce costs that fall within a broadened definition of quality. Examples include improved coordination of care for high-risk patients, variation reduction, and other forms of process improvement (also known as lean management). These forms of quality improvement are not captured by current publicly reported quality measures, but they are important focuses for provider organizations. Indeed, these types of work cannot be undertaken unless providers are well organized.

Market Forces Can Control Costs

For every provider who hopes costs can be contained through better quality, there is probably at least one health care purchaser who believes that "unleashing market forces" will drive waste out of health care and raise the quality. The ways in which these market forces would be unleashed include exposing patients to the true costs of care and providing data on the value (i.e., the quality and costs) of care for various providers.

There are two crucial limitations to this approach. First, patients do not particularly appreciate being exposed to costs, especially when they are sick. So people are not signing up in large numbers for health plan products that seek to turn them into consumers. Second, the data to help patients make choices are just not that helpful. They are difficult to understand and do not seem to address many issues about which many patients care, such as access to the latest technologies and experts on the cutting-edge of their fields.

We do believe that public reporting exerts a healthy pressure on providers and that patients need incentives to participate in efforts to mitigate increases in costs. Tiered pharmacy formularies in which patients pay low co-payments (e.g., $5 to $10) for generic medications, midrange co-payments (e.g., $20 to $25) for preferred brand-name drugs, and high co-payments ($50 or more) for nonpreferred drugs have been successful in reducing pharmacy spending without detectable adverse effects for patient care. Can this approach be applied to hospitals or physicians with greater benefit than harm? Time will tell.

A Single-Payer System Would Address All Our Problems

For every political conservative who hopes that market forces can solve health care's woes, there is a counterpart on the ideological Left who believes that a single government-run health care system would do the same. Advocates point to countries such as Canada and the United Kingdom where single-payer systems provide access to all citizens, and where the populations enjoy health that is as good as or better than in the United States.

A single-payer system could address the issue of access to health insurance for all Americans. The U.S. culture is less trusting of government to solve major social challenges than that of other countries, however, so the development of a single-payer system still seems unlikely in the foreseeable future. That said, the disruptive impact of so many Americans without insurance or whose insurance does not cover them adequately could lead to a much larger role for government in health care in the future.

Even if a single-payer system develops in the United States, it would not necessarily address the quality and safety problems generated by a fragmented delivery system, unless it changes reimbursement with the goal of encouraging the organization of providers. Medicare and Medicaid currently pay most doctors and hospitals on a fee-for-service basis, and at a lower rate than most commercial insurance plans. The result is that providers have incentives to do more and more, not better and better.

Physicians' Individual Autonomy Is the Most Important Guarantee of Quality

Saving the most uncomfortable myth for last, we now offer a direct challenge to physician colleagues who oppose any compromise of their individual autonomy. These physicians argue that medicine is a mix of art and science, and that evidence-based guidelines cannot dictate the right thing to do in every situation. They look with scorn on "cookbook medicine," and worry that any effort to control costs might do so at the expense of their patients' outcomes. They want to be free to do what is best for their patients, and make their own judgment about what that might be. They do not want to be forced to work in teams, and they do not want to be told what to do.

Many of the physicians who feel this way are, in fact, wonderful people and terrific doctors in a traditional sense. They work hard and they do their best for their patients—as individuals. They hover by the bedside when their patients are sick. In another era, these physicians represented the best that medicine could offer. The respect that these physicians earned and the autonomy that came with it *were* in fact the most important guarantees of quality.

But times have changed in two critical ways. First, rising costs shine a spotlight on the tremendous unexplainable variation in care patterns among physicians—raising the question of whether they can *all* be practicing the best medicine. Efforts to reduce variation inevitably erode individual physician autonomy.

Second, the explosion of knowledge means that much more is known about what is beneficial for patients, and makes possible increased roles for nonphysicians in the delivery of care. Nurses, pharmacists, and even the patients themselves can be active participants in health care delivery, if physicians will let them be members of the team. For those teams to be effective, everyone—including physicians—has to use the same playbooks. That means following the same protocols, using the same terminology, and updating teammates on what is happening. And being part of a team inevitably means giving up some autonomy—that is, if you want your team to win.

There are still countless opportunities when the right thing to do is unknown, when physicians need to use their creativity and test multiple ideas in the search for a strategy that will help their patients. We think physician autonomy will always be a key value in medicine.

But individual physician autonomy is not the *highest* value in medicine, and there are times when it should be placed subservient to other values—most notably what is best for patients. Many patients are better off if they receive care from teams that include nonphysicians. We think these patients include the sick ones, the healthy ones, the ones with chronic diseases, and the ones with complex medical conditions. In short, virtually all patients can benefit from the work of teams that provide care to them outside the physician office visit.

If physicians do not participate in such teams, the gap tends to get filled by health insurance plans. These insurance plans turn to carve-out companies that often call patients directly on the telephone to inquire whether they have had flu shots, are feeling well, and so on. These companies usually do not involve the physician at all, and when they do try to communicate with patients' doctors, many physicians refuse to answer their calls.

In this common context, physicians may think they have preserved their individual autonomy, but the result is a fragmentation of care, and a diminution of the roles of physicians and other providers. James Reinertsen has argued that physicians face a Zen-like paradox in which they must surrender some individual autonomy in order to preserve autonomy for the profession as a whole [4].

The Coevolution of Payment and Providers

Aware that in the last section we may have offended advocates for consumers and quality improvement, conservatives and liberals, and our own physician colleagues, we now call on them to work together to create an environment that accelerates the evolution of the health care delivery system. Let's return to the figure showing the relationship between payment methodologies and the state of provider organization, and the rough correlation between them. The diagonal line defines the comfort zone in which provider organization and payment methodology are matched. The horizontal bars describe some of the types of systems that providers adopt as they move toward the upper right of the figure.

The question for this final chapter is not how to match a payment system to a stage of provider evolution, but how to accelerate evolution so that providers organize more quickly and can accept new payment methodologies more rapidly. We are painfully aware of the unhappiness among providers generated by any effort to drive them into more organized groups and any change in the payment system that puts them at greater risk for the costs of care. Nevertheless, we believe that accelerated movement toward the upper right of this figure is critical to meeting the challenges of our times.

We are not at all sure that migration *all* the way to upper right is possible or even desirable, as long as patients continue to demand freedom to seek care from providers outside of specified networks. The reason: no one wants to hold financial risk that they cannot control. As long as most patients are in insurance products that allow them the freedom to fragment their care, providers holding the financial risk for their care will wonder about the sustainability of their contractual

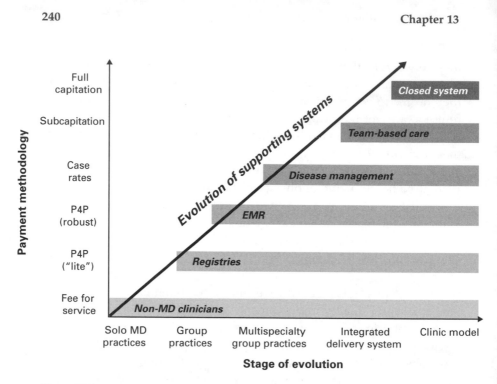

Figure 13.1
Evolving reimbursement and care models. P4P = pay for performance; EMR = electronic
medical records. (Reproduced with permission from TH Lee and RA Berenson, "The
Organization of Health Care Delivery: A Roadmap for Accelerated Improvement," in *The
Health Care Delivery System* [Washington, DC: Center for American Progress, 2008],
available at <http://www.americanprogress.org/issues/2008/10/pdf/health_delivery
_full.pdf>)

arrangement, and look to exit that arrangement after the first or second
bad year. We would thus be surprised if most of U.S. health care
approaches the model of a fully integrated clinic caring for patients
under capitation in the next decade or so.

Still, meaningful progress in quality and efficiency can be accomplished through the accelerated coevolution of payment and providers.
We say coevolution because major movement on either the x- or y-axis
of the figure is unlikely to be successful without corresponding movement on the other. A combination of payment carrots and sticks can be
used to nudge providers into organized groups that can accept increasing accountability for quality and efficiency.

A plausible "escalation strategy" might be:

1. Major payers announce that there will be minimal or no increases
for pure fee-for-service care—ever again. In other words, increases in

funding that would have been used to cover inflation in provider costs in the past will be used to reward better performance in the future. This approach sounds radical, but it is far from theoretical; after all, Medicare has been giving hospitals and physicians annual increases that fall short of consumer price inflation for several consecutive years now. To soften the blow if other payers implement this approach, the date at which the permanent freeze goes into effect could be put off by two to three years to allow providers time to make appropriate plans, or providers might be allowed annual increases that fall short of consumer price inflation.

2. Payers offer a flexible payment approach in which greater financial risk is accompanied by greater potential rewards. For example, physicians might get increases that correspond to consumer price inflation (e.g., 3 percent) if they achieve specified quality targets, but could get increases consistent with medical inflation (e.g., 5 to 6 percent) if they also achieve efficiency targets for pharmaceutical prescribing and radiology test ordering. (Medical inflation tends to be 2 to 3 percent higher than consumer price inflation, because hospitals and doctors have to invest in more advanced technologies and information systems each year, and because nursing salaries have risen faster than other labor costs.)

3. To achieve margins beyond medical inflation, providers would have to be sufficiently organized to accept payments like the medical home and bundled case rates. Under these payment systems, providers might just break even financially if they were providing unexceptional care with unexceptional complication rates. But if providers were effective, efficient, and creative in their care, they could share in the substantial savings that result from averted hospitalizations.

4. The greatest financial rewards might be earned by provider organizations that were sufficiently organized and had sufficient confidence in their ability to manage their patient population to accept capitation. These rewards would not be greater because of higher budgets for these patient populations but rather because providers taking responsibility for the totality of care have more opportunities to find ways to improve efficiency.

We emphasize again that we are not arguing for a relentless drive of providers into clinics that are paid through capitation. For reasons described above, we are concerned about the sustainability of capitation when patients have freedom to choose providers outside their main provider network. Capitation will always have to deal with tensions about whether the budget is sufficient to provide good care and whether there is a reasonable chance for reward (greater than fifty-fifty) to providers who assume the risk. Uncertainty surrounds issues as fundamental as who decides whether a capitation budget is adequate for high-quality care and whether patients should have the right to purchase more care with their own resources.

That said, we think that any movement toward the upper right will be beneficial for patients and the health care system. By holding fee-for-service payments below the level of inflation, Medicare and Medicaid have already created the stick; we are contending that these government payers and commercial insurers should create the carrots that encourage providers to move more rapidly along the road of greater organization. In the final section of this chapter and book, we describe the roles of the various stakeholders that will help accelerate movement in that direction.

Roles for Stakeholders

The stakeholders in health care who can collectively accelerate the evolution of health care include health insurance plans, employers, patients, government policymakers—and of course providers themselves. All of these groups have considerable influence over the pace of change. All of them have the ability to slow change down when their fear of the unknown exceeds the pain of the status quo. But if they share a common vision of what a better health care system might look like, these stakeholders can collaborate to speed its development.

Our argument throughout this book has been that any vision of a better health care system must include more integrated care delivered by more organized providers. Various stakeholders may differ on the potential role of the patient-consumer as a market force putting pressure on providers to improve or as the actual organizers of their own care. But stakeholders who share the belief that more integrated care is a worthy goal should step back and consider whether their policies are speeding or slowing the organization of providers. Our recommendation is that all stakeholders should include greater organization of providers in their visions for health care's future. The policies and actions that logically flow from such a shared vision are numerous; some are described below.

Public Reporting

Current performance measures that are publicly reported help drive "microsystem" improvement, such as what an individual doctor does when seeing a patient with diabetes. We need "macrosystem" improvement, which is more likely to be driven by measures that go across entire episodes of patients' care.

Accordingly, organizations that publicly report on provider performance should consider whether current measures that were developed for a fragmented health care system should be augmented by measures that reflect the effectiveness of integration of care by organized providers. Examples of measures of integration might include the:

• Percentage of physicians using an EMR (so that clinicians can see each other's notes)

• Percentage of prescriptions written by computer (so that decision support can guide clinicians to the safest and most efficient choices, and so that other clinicians can be clear on just what the patient is taking)

• Percentage of hospitalized patients with heart failure who are triaged into an outpatient heart failure program prior to discharge (so that optimal care for the patient does not stop when they move from one part of the health care system to another)

• Reliability of flow of accurate medication lists when patients are discharged from hospitals to home or other levels of care

Many health care providers are not sufficiently organized to even measure their performance according to such "systemness" parameters. We think that these measures of integration could be more valuable drivers of progress than measures of what individual physicians and individual hospitals do. Our patients seem less interested in publicly reported measures on our reliability in testing control levels in diabetics than the fact that our doctors know what each other are doing through our EMR.

There are other implications for public reporting initiatives if their true primary targets are providers in general and provider organizations in particular. Our recommendations are that these initiatives focus on quality rather than efficiency, recognizing the doubts that public reporting on cost has any beneficial effects. And when physicians are organized into groups, we recommend that most quality data should be reported at the physician group level, rather than for individual physicians.

We recognize that consumers are more interested in data on individual physicians, but the methodological challenges of accumulating an adequate sample size for individual doctors and then adjusting for differences in the severity of illness are huge. The risk of misclassification of individual physicians is high, and as a result, physicians tend to be angered by the process and dismissive of the results—not a great starting point for stimulating earnest efforts to improve.

On the other hand, quality data that are reported for groups of physicians are less emotionally charged for doctors, more likely to be statistically valid, and also more likely to describe a unit of organization that can initiate improvement efforts. We *would*, however, favor giving those provider groups data on the performance of their individual physicians for use in internal improvement efforts. The level of methodological rigor required by physicians for such data is not as high when the physicians do not feel at risk of public humiliation or exclusion from insurance products.

Payers and Employers

From a financial perspective, health insurance plans and employers have much to gain but substantial risk from greater provider organization. The danger is that organized providers will negotiate more effectively than fragmented providers. If contract negotiations are solely about the price that is paid for various clinical services, higher payment rates would obviously translate into higher overall health care costs.

On the other hand, organized providers have the ability to sign contracts in which they are accountable for more than performing office visits and caring for patients during hospitalizations. Payers and employers should thus adopt the flexible payment strategy described earlier in this chapter, in which the potential financial rewards are greater for providers if they assume greater risk for quality and cost. Health insurance plans (including Medicare and Medicaid) should offer several options for payment to providers, but it should be obvious that more organized provider groups have a good chance of financial success if they deliver high-quality and efficient care. The solo physician who wants to maintain complete autonomy should have the right to do so, but that physician should understand that his or her business model does not have bright prospects.

In summary, we recommend a flexible contracting structure that explicitly rewards the integration of care by organized providers. We urge payers and employers to pursue this approach rather than focus on the shifting of costs to patients. In an upcoming section, we will describe what providers must do to make this approach viable.

Patients

Patients can accelerate the evolution of health care by articulating what they really want and then demanding it. These demands should include:

• Access to physicians who are polite and knowledgeable as individuals, but who also know what other physicians are doing and saying

• The ability to interact with their physicians' practices outside of business hours for information and routine services such as scheduling appointments, renewing prescriptions, and arranging referrals

• The availability of teams and programs that help them stay healthy and reduce the risk of complications of their medical conditions

And that is just for starters.

Organized groups of providers are more likely to be able to deliver the kind of integration that can make health care much better for patients. We are quite aware that large provider groups have not always provided the warm personal services of small physician practices, where the office staff might recognize patients as soon as they walk in the door. Indeed, patient satisfaction tends to be lower for care delivered by larger provider organizations, where patients may not feel that they have one doctor who is focused on their interests.

We do not think that patients should have to choose between personalized and integrated care, though. Organized providers can learn to offer care with personalized warmth, but we doubt that most one or two physician practices can adopt the systems needed to coordinate and improve care. The physicians in these small practices are just as smart and hardworking as their colleagues in larger organizations, but the business case for them to invest in such systems is weaker, and the costs are higher. So we would encourage patients to ask for what they really want and then look to see if organized provider groups can offer it.

Policymakers

We have three major requests for government policymakers. First, we ask that policymakers recognize that the potential benefits from provider organization are considerable, and that the risks to the consumer from greater provider negotiating effectiveness can be managed. The traditional philosophy of the Federal Trade Commission and other government agencies has been to promote competition among providers as the surest way to improve quality and hold down costs.

The fear has been that providers would form cartels that would extract higher payment rates without creating any actual increase in the value in return. In this context, there has been suspicion that organized providers were a threat to the consumer. The result has been numerous policies that have the unintended effect of suppressing delivery system innovation [5].

Competition *is* healthy for health care, but collaboration among providers is essential for many of the types of improvements described in this book, and we think there is a middle ground in which competition and collaboration can coexist. The Federal Trade Commission is actively exploring that middle ground, and has defined "clinical integration" as a legal framework in which health care providers can collaborate to improve quality and efficiency, and negotiate contracts together even if they are not members of a single business entity. That work strikes us as worthwhile and should continue.

The second request of government policymakers is to consider a major investment in the information infrastructure of health care. Although our own organization has been able to fund CPOE in the hospitals and EMRs for our physicians, most providers have not. These hospitals and physician practices simply do not know how they will be able to raise the funds for needed information technology at a time when payments from Medicare and Medicaid fall short of their actual costs, and when commercial insurers have little interest in paying for such infrastructure. A logical and appropriate role of government is to provide funding for health care information systems—with the condition that providers support interoperability among their electronic records, so that patient information is available when and where it is needed. The 2009 Obama administration economic stimulus package is a major step in the right direction; undoubtedly, additional steps will be needed in future years.

The third request is for government to support and fund a federal program to perform analyses of the comparative effectiveness of high-cost drugs and technology. This program could be modeled after the United Kingdom's National Institute for Health and Clinical Excellence, which provides guidance on the use of technologies and other areas of clinical practice. If a single highly respected group can develop authoritative recommendations for how drugs and technologies should be used, then organized providers can put in place systems to ensure that the recommendations are followed.

The Obama administration also plans major investments in such "effectiveness review." It may take years to learn how to get the greatest impact from this work. We hope the government, providers, and the rest of the health care community will be patient and will collaborate in this effort.

Providers

The requirements for providers are difficult but clear. If providers are not part of an organization that can implement systems to improve quality and efficiency, they should join one. If none exists around them, they should form one. If they are part of a provider organization, they should ask what they can do to make it more effective.

The status quo is not viable for the purchasers of health care and it is not working that well for patients either. It is only a matter of time until the pressure for change on providers increases so that it is unbearable. Providers should shape the change instead of just reacting to it.

Providers should actively participate in public reporting efforts, not resist them. From a purely practical perspective, public reporting is here to stay, and it is a foolish waste of political capital to oppose it. From a more idealistic perspective, providers should concede that public reporting has the potential to exert a healthy pressure for improvements in quality. Accordingly, providers should seek invitations to the tables at which public reporting initiatives are planned, and once there, dispel any notions that they are there to protect their colleagues from scrutiny.

Physicians and other providers should ask themselves what kind of systems (e.g., registries, EMRs, or disease management programs) they should implement with the goal of improving quality and efficiency. The real reason to implement these systems is to make care for their patients better, but an acid test is whether these systems enable the provider group to consider payment forms that are more prospective. If providers invest in such systems, there should be a reward so that at the very least, the providers break even financially.

To get access to these rewards, providers will have to be open to new payment methodologies that will require taking greater risk than fee for service. As managers with fiduciary responsibilities for our own organization, we fully understand how nerve-racking it is to change payment models and take on risk for issues not fully within our control. But we are certain that fighting off alternatives to fee for service is an even riskier strategy. We providers and the other stakeholders in health care need to experiment with and learn how to implement other payment models, and how to disseminate their successes widely.

Our final recommendation is that provider leaders take on the cultural challenges. They should make unambiguous their belief that physicians are not just providers of services to individual patients but that they also should be stewards of the health care system itself. As such, physicians have obligations to use resources efficiently, participate in efforts to make health care better financially viable, and play their role on teams that coordinate and improve care. Physicians should be supportive of exploration of such innovations, as long as there is a realistic prospect that they be beneficial for patients.

A better, less chaotic, higher quality health care system is within our reach—if physicians and other health care stakeholders work together to organize and integrate care.

References

Chapter 1: Chaos

1. Committee on Quality of Health Care in America, Institute of Medicine. *To Err Is Human: Building a Safer Health System*. Washington, DC: National Academy Press, 2000.

2. Committee on Quality of Health Care in America, Institute of Medicine. *Crossing the Quality Chasm: A New Health System for the 21st Century*. Washington, DC: National Academy Press, 2001.

3. McGlynn EA, Asch SM, Adams J, et al. The quality of health care delivered to adults in the United States. *N Engl J Med* 2003;348:2635–2645.

4. Asch SM, Kerr EA, Keesey J, et al. Who is at greatest risk for receiving poor-quality health care? *N Engl J Med* 2006;354:1147–1156.

5. Schoen C, Davis K, How SKH, Schoenbaum SC. U.S. health system performance: A national scorecard. *Health Aff* 2006:w457–w475.

6. *Commonwealth Fund Commission on a High Performance Health System. Why Not the Best? Results from the National Scorecard on U.S. Health System Performance, 2008*. Available at <http://www.commonwealthfund.org/publications/publications_show.htm?doc_id=692682> (accessed July 29, 2008).

7. McGlynn EA. *Assessing the Appropriateness of Care: How Much Is Too Much?* RAND Research Brief. Santa Monica, CA: RAND, 1998. Available at <http://www.rand.org/pubs/research_briefs/RB4522> (accessed March 6, 2009).

8. Blendon RJ, DesRoches CM, Brodie M, et al. Views of practicing physicians and the public on medical errors. *N Engl J Med* 2002;347:1933–1940.

9. Dunn J, Lee TH, Percelay JM, Fitz JG, Goldman L. Patient and house officer attitudes on physician attire and etiquette. *JAMA* 1987;257:65–68.

10. Available at <http://www.nlm.nih.gov/bsd/bsd_key.html> (accessed July 29, 2008).

11. Desroches CM, Campbell EG, Rao SR, et al. Electronic health records in ambulatory care—a national survey of physicians. *N Engl J Med* 2008;359:50–60.

12. Garibaldi RA, Popkave C, BylsmaW. Career plans for trainees in internal medicine residency programs. *Acad Med* 2005;80:507–512.

13. Association of American Medical Colleges. *Medical Student Education: Cost, Debt, and Resident Stipend Facts.* Available at <http://www.aamc.org/students/financing/debthelp/factcard05.pdf> (accessed January 15, 2007).

14. Dorsey ER, Jarjoura D, Rutecki GW. Influence of controllable lifestyle on recent trends in specialty choice by US medical students. *JAMA* 2003;290:1173–1178.

15. Bond JT, Thompson C, Galinsky E, Prottas D. *The 2002 National Study of the Changing Workforce.* New York: Families and Work Institute, 2002.

16. Fogg N, Harrington P, Kochan TA. *The State of Working Families in Massachusetts.* Work-Family Council Initiative Working Paper Series, January 2004. Available at <http://web.mit/edue/workplacecenter/docs/WFI-WPS.pdf> (accessed January 18, 2007).

17. Poon EG, Gandhi TK, Sequist TD, Murff HJ, Karson AS, Bates DW. "I wish I had seen this test result earlier!" Dissatisfaction with test result management systems in primary care. *Arch Intern Med* 2004;164:2223–2228.

18. Poon EG, Wang SJ, Gandhi TK, Bates DW, Kuperman GJ. Design and implementation of a comprehensive outpatient results manager. *J Biomed Inform* 2003;36:80–91.

19. St. Peter RF, Reed MC, Kemper P, Blumenthal D. Changes in the scope of care provided by primary care physicians. *N Engl J Med* 1999;341:1980–1985.

20. Smith PC, Araya R, Bublitz C, et al. Missing clinical information during primary care visits. *JAMA* 2005;293:565–571.

21. Yarnall KS, et al. Primary care: Is there enough time for prevention? *Am J Public Health* 2003;93:635.

22. Ostbye T, et al. Is there time for management of patients with chronic disease in primary care? *Ann Fam Med* 2005;3:209.

23. Gurwitz JH, Field TS, Harrold LR, et al. Incidence and preventability of adverse drug events among older persons in the ambulatory setting. *JAMA* 2003;289:1107–1116.

24. Available at <http://www.cnn.com/exchange/ireports/topics/forms/2007/01/saving.your.life.html> (accessed January 18, 2007).

25. Hampton T. Flawed prescribing practices revealed. *JAMA* 2006;296:2191–1292.

26. Prescosolido BA, Tuch SA, Martin JK. The profession of medicine and the public. *J Health Soc Behav* 2001;42:1–16.

27. Mechanic D, McAlpine DD, Rosenthal M. Are patients' office visits with physicians getting shorter? *N Engl J Med* 2001;344:198–204.

28. *Commonwealth Fund Survey of Public Views of the U.S. Health Care System, 2008.* Available at <http://www.commonwealthfund.org/surveys/surveys_show.htm?doc_id=698589> (accessed August 9, 2008).

29. *Commonwealth Fund International Health Policy Survey, 2002.* Available at <http://www.commonwealthfund.org/surveys/surveys_show.htm?doc_id=228168> (accessed August 9, 2008).

30. Safran DG. Defining the future of primary care: What can we learn from patients? *Ann Intern Med* 2003;138:248–255.

31. Wilson IB, Schoen C, Neuman P, et al. Physician-patient communication about prescription nonadherence: A 50–state study of America's seniors. *J Gen Intern Med* 2007.

Chapter 2: Progress

1. Davis K, Schoen C, Guterman S, Shih T, Schoenbaum SC, Weinbaum I. *Slowing the Growth of U.S. Health Care Expenditures: What Are the Options?* New York: Commonwealth Fund, January 2007.

2. Congressional Budget Office. *Technological Change and the Growth of Health Care Spending.* CBO Paper. Available at <http://www.cbo.gov/ftpdocs/89xx/doc8947/01-31-Tech-Health.pdf> (accessed July 30, 2008).

3. Zukerman S, McFeeters J. *Recent Growth in Health Expenditures.* New York: Commonwealth Fund, March 2006. Available at <http://www.cmwf.org/publications/publications_show.htm?doc_id=362803> (accessed February 18, 2007).

4. PricewaterhouseCoopers for America's Health Insurance Plans. *The Factors Fueling Rising Healthcare Costs 2006.* February 2006.

5. Strunk BC, Ginsburg PB, Banker MI. The effect of population aging on future hospital demand. *Health Affairs* 2006;25:w141–w149.

6. Bodenheimer T. Health and rising health care costs. Part 1: Seeking an explanation. *Ann Intern Med* 2005;142:847–854.

7. Legorreta AP, Silber JH, Costantino GN, Kobylinski RW, Zatz SL. Increased cholecystectomy rate after the introduction of laparoscopic cholecystectomy. *JAMA* 1993;270:1429–1432.

8. Altman KL. So many advances in medicine, so many yet to come. *New York Times.* December 26, 2006. Available at <http://query.nytimes.com/gst/fullpage.html?res=9503E7DC1E31F935A15751C1A9609C8B63> (accessed March 7, 2009).

9. Walensky RP, Paltiel AD, Losina E, et al. The survival benefits of AIDS treatment in the United States. *J Infect Dis* 2006;194:11–19.

10. Nathan DM. Finding new treatments for diabetes—how many, how fast . . . how good? *N Engl J Med* 2007;356:437–440.

11. Fox KAA, Gabriel P, Eagle KA, et al. Decline in rates of death and heart failure in acute coronary syndromes, 1999–2006. *JAMA* 2007;297:1892–1900.

12. The REST Investigators. Uterine-artery embolization versus surgery for symptomatic uterine fibroids. *N Engl J Med* 2007:356:360–370.

13. Lynch TJ, Bell DW, Sordella R, et al. Activating mutations in the epidermal growth factor receptor underlying responsiveness of non-small-cell lung cancer to gefitinib. *N Engl J Med* 2004;350:2129–2139.

14. McClellan MB. Technology and innovation: Their effects on cost growth of healthcare. Testimony before the Joint Economic Committee of the U.S. Congress. July 9, 2003. Available at http://www.fda.gov/ola/2003/healthcare0709.html> (accessed March 7, 2009).

15. Schackman BR, Gebo KA, Walensky RP, et al. The lifetime cost of current human immunodeficiency virus care in the United States. *Med Care* 2006;44:990–997.

16. Cutler DM. *Your Money or Your Life: Strong Medicine for America's Health Care System.* New York: Oxford University Press, 2004.

17. Meltzer MI. Health economics and prioritising health care. *Lancet* 2008;372:612–613.

18. McGlynn EA, Asch SM, Adams J, et al. The quality of health care delivered to adults in the United States. *N Engl J Med* 2003;348:2635–2664.

Chapter 3: Fragmentation

1. Pham HH, Schrag D, O'Malley AS, Wu B, Bach PB. Care patterns in Medicare and their implications for pay for performance. *N Engl J Med* 2007;356:1130–1139.

2. Orszag PR. The overuse, underuse, and misuse of health care. Testimony before the Committee on Finance, U.S. Senate. June 17, 2008. Available at <http://www.cbo.gov> (accessed August 9, 2008).

3. Fisher, ES, et al. The implications of regional variations in Medicare spending, part 2: Health outcomes and satisfaction with care. *Ann Intern Med* 2003;138:288–298.

4. Wennberg JE, Fisher ES, Skinner JS. Geography and the debate over Medicare reform. *Health Aff* 2002:w96–w97.

5. Horwitz JR. Making profits and providing care: Comparing nonprofit, for-profit, and government hospitals. *Health Aff* 2005;24:790–801.

6. Hing E, Cherry DK, Woodwell DA. National Ambulatory Medical Care Survey: 2004 summary. *CDC Advance Data* 2006:374. Available at <http://www.cdc.gov/nchs/data/ad/ad374.pdf>.

7. Wigton RS, Alguire P. The declining number and variety of procedures done by general internists: A resurvey of members of the American College of Physicians. *Ann Intern Med* 2007;146:355–360.

8. Bodenheimer T. Coordinating care: A perilous journey through the health care system. *N Engl J Med* 2008;358:1064–1071.

9. Kripalani S, LeFevre F, Phillips CO, Williams MV, Basaviah P, Baker DW. Deficits in communication and information transfer between hospital-based and primary care physicians: Implications for patient safety and continuity of care. *JAMA* 2007;297:831–841.

10. Berenson RA, Ginsburg PB, May JH. Hospital-physician relations: Cooperation, competition, or separation. *Health Aff* 2007;26:w31–w43.

11. Goldsmith J. Hospitals and physicians: Not a pretty picture. *Health Aff* 2007;26:w72–w75.

12. Guyatt G, Cairns J, Churchill D, et al. Evidence-based medicine: A new approach to teaching the practice of medicine. *JAMA* 1992;268:2420–2425.

13. Medicare Payment Advisory Commission. Report to Congress. *Reforming the Delivery System.* Available at <http://www.medpac.gov/documents/Jun08_EntireReport.pdf> (accessed August 3, 2008).

Chapter 4: What Does Organization in Health Care Look Like?

1. Ketcham JD, Baker LC, MacIsaac D. Physician practice size and variations in treatment and outcomes: Evidence from Medicare patients with AMI. *Health Aff* 2007;26:195–205.

2. Audet AM, Doty MM, Shamasdin J, Schoenbaum SC. Measure, learn, and improve: Physician's involvement in quality improvement. *Health Aff* 2005;24:843–853.

3. Pham HH, Schrag D, Hargraves JL, et al. Delivery of preventive services to older adults by primary care physicians. *JAMA* 2005;294:473–481.

4. Friedberg MW, Cotlin KL, Pearson SD, et al. Does affiliation of physician groups with one another produce higher quality primary care? *J Gen Intern Med* 2007;22:1385–1392.

5. Li P, Bahensky JA, Jaana M, Ward MM. Role of multihospital system membership in electronic medical record adoption. *Health Care Manage Rev* 2008;33:169–177.

6. Mehrotra A, Epstein AM, Rosenthal MB. Do integrated medical groups provide higher quality medical care than individual practice associations? *Ann Intern Med* 2006;145:826–833.

7. McMenamin S, et al. Health promotion in physician organizations: Results from a national study. *Am J Prev Med* 2004;26:259–264.

8. Gilles RR, Chenok KE, Shortell SM, et al. The impact of health plan delivery system organization on clinical quality and patient satisfaction. *Health Services Research* 2006;41:1181–1199.

9. Lee TH. Eulogy for a quality measure. *N Engl J Med* 2007;357:1175–1177.

10. Beta-Blocker Heart Attack (BHAT) investigators: A randomized trial of propranolol in patients with acute myocardial infarction. I. Mortality results. *JAMA* 1982;247: 1707–1714.

11. Gottlieb SS, Marcarter RJ, Vogel RA. Effect of beta-blockade on mortality among high-risk and low-risk patients after myocardial infarction. *N Engl J Med* 1998;339:489–497.

12. Lamas GA, Pfeffer MA, Hamm P, Wertheimer J, Rouleau JL, Braunwald E. Do the results of randomized clinical trials of cardiovascular drugs influence medical practice? The SAVE investigators. *N Engl J Med* 1992;327:241–247.

13. Braunwald E., ed. *Heart Disease: A Textbook of Cardiovascular Medicine.* 2nd ed. Philadelphia: W. B. Saunders, 1984.

14. Burwen DR, Galusha DH, Lewis JM, et al. National and state trends in quality of care for acute myocardial infarction between 1994–1995 and 1998–1999. *Arch Intern Med* 2003;163:1430–1439.

15. Lindenauer PK, Remus D, Roman S, et al. Public reporting and pay for performance in hospital quality improvement. *N Engl J Med* 2007;356:486–496.

16. Available at <http://www.acc.org/qualityandscience/gap/gap_program.htm> (accessed August 4, 2008).

17. Available at <http://www.americanheart.org/presenter.jhtml?identifier=3045578> (accessed August 4, 2008).

18. Available at <http://www.ihi.org/ihi/Programs/campaign/campaign.htm?tabid=1> (accessed on August 4, 2008).

19. The Commonwealth Fund Commission on a High Performance Health System. Why Not the Best? Results from the National Scorecard on U.S. Health System Performance, September 2006. Available at <http://www.commonwealthfund.org/usr_doc/Commission_whynotthebest_951.pdf?section=4039> (accessed August 4, 2008).

20. The Commonwealth Fund Commission on a High Performance Health System. Why Not the Best? Results from the National Scorecard on U.S. Health System Performance, 2008. Available at <http://www.commonwealthfund.org/publications/publications_show.htm?doc_id=692682> (accessed July 29, 2008).

21. Committee on Quality of Health Care in America, Institute of Medicine. *Crossing the Quality Chasm: A New Health System for the 21st Century.* Washington, DC: National Academy Press, 2001.

Chapter 5: What Kinds of Systems Improve Health Care?

1. See <http://web.ncqa.org/tabid/141/Default.aspx> (accessed September 3, 2007).

2. Congressional Budget Office. Evidence on the costs and benefits of health information technology. Congressional Budget Office Paper, May 2008. Available at <http://www.cbo .gov/ftpdocs/95xx/doc9572/07–24–HealthIT.pdf> (accessed on August 7, 2008).

3. Blumenthal D, Glaser JP. Information technology comes to medicine. *N Engl J Med* 2007;356:2527–2534.

4. Desroches CM, Campbell EG, Rao SR, et al. Electronic health records in ambulatory care: A national survey of physicians. *N Engl J Med* 2008;359:50–60.

5. Girosi F, Meili R, Scoville R. *Extrapolating Evidence of Health Information Technology Savings and Costs.* Santa Monica, CA: RAND Corporation, 2005. Available at <http://www.rand.org/pubs/monographs/2005/RAND_MG410.sum.pdf> (accessed August 9, 2008).

6. Hillestad R, Bigelow J, Bower A, et al. Can electronic medical record systems transform health care? Potential health benefits, savings, and costs. *Health Aff* 2005; 24:1103–1117.

7. Pan E, et al. *The Value of Healthcare Information Exchange and Interoperability.* Wellesley, MA: Center for Information Technology Leadership, 2004.

8. Walker J, Pan E, Johnson D, Adler-Milstein J, Bates DW, Middleton B. The value of health care information exchange and interoperability. *Health Aff* 2005;25:w5–10–w5–18.

9. Garrido T, Jamieson L, Zhou Y, Wiesenthal A, Liang L. Effect of electronic health records in ambulatory care: Retrospective, serial, cross sectional study. *British Med J* 2005;330:581–585.

10. Kaushal R, Shojania KG, Bates DW. Effects of computerized physician order entry and clinical decision systems on medication safety: A systematic review. *Arch Intern Med* 2003;163:1409–1416.

11. Koppel R, Metlay JP, Cohen A, et al. Role of computerized physician order entry systems in facilitating medication errors. *JAMA* 2005;293:1197–1203.

12. Bodenheimer T, Wagner EH, Grumbach K. Improving primary care for patients with chronic illness. *JAMA* 2002;288:1775–1779.

13. Bodenheimer T, Wagner EH, Grumbach K. Improving primary care for patients with chronic illness: The chronic care model, part 2. *JAMA* 2002;288:1909–1914.

14. Mattke S, Seid M, Mai S. Evidence for the effect of disease management: Is $1 billion a year a good investment? *Am J Manag Care* 2007;13:670–676.

15. Casalino LP. Disease management and the organization of physician practice. *JAMA* 2005;293:485–488.

Chapter 6: Tightly Structured Health Care Delivery Organizations

1. Available at <http://www.va.gov/OCA/testimony/hvac/sh/kizer724.asp> (accessed March 1, 2009).

2. Available at <http://www.va.gov/OCA/testimony/svac/22SE9810.asp> (accessed March 1, 2009).

3. Jonathan Perlin, personal communication.

4. Available at <https://acsnsqip.org/main/about_history.asp> (accessed August 9, 2008).

5. Perlin J. Quality outcomes of the performance management program in "the new VHA." *Monitor* 2000;5:11–17.

6. Petersen LA, Normand S-LT, Daley J, McNeil BJ. Outcome of myocardial infarction in Veterans Health Administration patients as compared with Medicare patients. *N Engl J Med* 2000;343:1934–1941.

7. Jha AK, Perlin JB, Kizer KW, Dudley RA. Effect of the transformation of the Veterans Affairs Health Care system on the quality of care. *N Engl J Med* 2003;348:2218–2227.

8. Stewart AT, Raman AP. Lessons from Toyota's long drive. *Harvard Business Review* July–August 2007:74–83.

9. Connolly C. Toyota assembly lines inspire improvements at hospital. *Washington Post* June 3, 2005, A1.

10. Virginia Mason Medical Center Annual Report—2007. Available at <https://www.virginiamason.org/home/blank.cfm?xyzpdqabc=0&id=156&action=list&limit_issue=32> (accessed August 9, 2008).

11. Pham HH, Ginsburg PB, McKenzie K, Milstein A. Redesigning care delivery in response to a high performance network: Case study of the Virginia Mason Medical Center. *Health Aff* 2007;26:w532–w544.

12. Abelson R. In bid for better care, surgery with a warranty. *New York Times* May 17, 2007, p. 1.

13. Lee TH. Pay for performance, version 2.0? *N Engl J Med* 2007;357:531–533.

14. Casale AS, Paulus RA, Selna MJ, et al. "ProvenCare SM": A provider-driven pay-for-performance program for acute episodic cardiac surgical care. *Ann Surg* 2007;246:613–623.

15. Diamond F. Kaiser's asthma outcomes will take your breath away. *Managed Care* 2005. Available at <http://www.managedcaremag.com/archives/0503/0503.kaiser_asthma.html> (accessed March 7, 2009).

Chapter 7: Organizing the Mainstream of U.S. Medicine

1. Kastor JA. *Mergers of Teaching Hospitals in Boston, New York, and Northern California.* Ann Arbor: University of Michigan Press, 2001.

2. Shortell SM, Casalino LP. Health care reform requires accountable care systems. *JAMA* 2008;300:95–97.

3. Lee TH, Mongan JJ. Are healthcare's problems incurable? One integrated delivery system's program for transforming its care. Brookings Institution, 2006. Available at <http://www.brook.edu/views/papers/20061215_lee.htm (accessed March 2, 2009).

4. Mongan JJ, Mechanic R, Lee TH. Transforming U.S. health care: Policy challenges affecting the integration and improvement of care. Brookings Institution, 2006. Available at <http://www.brook.edu/views/papers/20061215_mongan.htm (accessed March 2, 2009).

5. Kaushal R, Bates DW, Poon EG, Jha A, Blumenthal D. Functional gaps in attaining a national health information network. *Health Aff* 2005;24:1281–1289.

6. Bates DW, Leape LL, Cullen DJ, et al. Effect of computerized physician order entry and a team intervention on prevention of serious medication errors. *JAMA* 1998;280: 1311–1316.

7. Guerra A. Ante up. *Healthcare Informatics* February 2008. Available at <http://www .healthcare-informatics.com> (accessed August 10, 2008).

8. Bates DW, Miller EB, Cullen DJ, et al. Patient risk factors for adverse drug events in hospitalized patients. *Arch Intern Med* 1999;159:2553–2560.

9. Evans RS, Pestotnik SL, Classen DC, et al. A computer-assisted management program for antibiotics and other antiinfective agents. *N Engl J Med* 1998;338:232–238.

10. Bates DW. Using information technology to reduce rates of medication errors in hospitals. *BMJ* 2000;320:788–791.

11. Rich MW, Beckham V, Wittenberg C, et al. A multidisciplinary intervention to prevent readmission of elderly patients with congestive heart failure. *N Engl J Med* 1995;333: 1190–1195.

12. Available at <http://www.medicalhomeinfo.org/> (accessed August 10, 2008).

13. Beal AC, Doty MM, Hernandez SE, Shea KK, Davis K. Closing the Divide: The Commonwealth Fund 2006 Health Care Quality Survey. Available at <http://www .commonwealthfund.org/surveys/surveys_show.htm?doc_id=506847> (accessed on August 10, 2008).

14. Davis K, Schoenbaum SC, Audet AJ. A 2020 vision of patient-centered primary care. Commonwealth Fund. Available at <http://www.commonwealthfund.org/usr _doc/868_Davis_2020_patient-centered_care_JGIM_10–2005_.pdf?section=4039> (accessed August 10, 2008).

15. Fisher ES. Building a medical neighborhood for the medical home. *N Engl J Med* 2008;359:1202–1205.

16. Iglehart JK. No place like home: Testing a new model of care delivery. *N Engl J Med* 2008;359:1200–1202.

17. Paulus RA, Davis K, Steele GD. Continuous innovation in health care: Implications of the Geisinger experience. Health Aff 2008;27:1235–1245.

18. Berenson RA, Hammons T, Gans DN, et al. A house is not a home: Keeping patients at the center of practice redesign. *Health Aff* 2008;27:1219–1230.

19. Rittenhouse DR, Casalino KP, Gillies RR, Shortell SM, Lau B. Measuring the medical home infrastructure in large medical groups. *Health Aff* 2008;27:1246–1258.

Chapter 8: What Can Payers, Employers, and Patients Do?

1. Lee TH, Zapert K. Do high deductible health plans threaten quality of care? *N Engl J Med* 2005;353:1202–1204.

2. Drug Benefit Trends. November 2007, 450.

3. Mattke S, Seid M, Mai S. Evidence for the effect of disease management: Is $1 billion a year a good investment? *Am J Manag Care* 2007;13:670–676.

4. Wang PS, Simon GE, Avorn J, et al. Telephone screening, outreach, and care management for depressed workers and impact on clinical and work productivity outcomes: A randomized controlled trial. *JAMA* 2007;298:1401–1411.

5. Aboa-Eboule C, Brisson C, Maunsell E, et al. Job strain and risk of acute recurrent coronary heart disease events. *JAMA* 2007;298:1652–1660.

6. Rosenthal MB, Landon BE, Normand ST, Frank RG, Ahmad TS, Epstein AE. Employers' use of value-based purchasing strategies. *JAMA* 2007;298:2281–2288.

Chapter 10: Provider Change

1. Gallagher TH, Waterman AD, Ebers AG, Fraser VJ, Levinson W. Patients' and physicians' attitudes regarding the disclosure of medical errors. *JAMA* 2003;289:1001–1007.

2. Gallagher TH, Studdert D, Levinson W. Disclosing harmful medical errors to patients. *N Engl J Med* 2007;356:2713–2729.

3. Goldman L, Sayson R, Robbins S, et al. The value of the autopsy in three medical eras. *N Engl J Med* 1983;308:1000–1005.

4. Congressional Budget Office. *Geographic Variation in Health Care Spending* February 2008. Available at <http://www.cbo.gov> (accessed August 12, 2008).

5. Kanouse DE, Kallich J, Kahan JP. Dissemination of effectiveness and outcomes research. *Health Policy* 1995;34:167–192.

6. Congressional Budget Office. *Research on the Comparative Effectiveness of Medical Treatments: Issues and Options for an Expanded Federal Role.* Available at <http://www.cbo.gov> (accessed August 12, 2008).

7. Blumenthal D, Glaser JP. Information technology comes to medicine. *N Engl J Med* 2007;356:2527–2534.

8. Iglehart J. Medicare's declining payments to physicians. *N Engl J Med* 2002:346: 1924–1930.

9. Iglehart J. Medicaid revisited: Skirmishes over a Vast Public Enterprise. *N Engl J Med* 2007;356:734–740.

10. Kotter J. Leading change: Why transformation efforts fail. *Harvard Business Review* January 1, 2007. Available at <http://harvardbusinessonline.hbsp.harvard.edu/b01/en/common/item_detail.jhtml;jsessionid=DKOCDDFBMM1T4AKRGWCB5VQBKE0YOISW?id=R0701J&referral=2341> (accessed March 4, 2009).

11. Kahneman D, Tversky A. *Choices, Values, and Frames.* Cambridge: Cambridge University Press, 2000.

12. Poundstone W. *Prisoner's Dilemma.* New York: Doubleday, 1992.

13. Axelrod R. *The Evolution of Cooperation.* New York: Basic Books, 1985.

14. Liker J. *The Toyota Way.* New York: McGraw-Hill, 2004.

15. Lee TH, Shiba S, Wood RC. *Integrated Management Systems: A Practical Approach to Transforming Organizations.* New York: Wiley, 1999.

Chapter 11: Payment Change

1. Fisher ES, Staiger DO, Bynum JPW, Gottlieb DJ. Creating accountable care organizations: The extended hospital medical staff. *Health Aff* 2007;26:w44–w57.

2. Shortell SM, Casolino LP. Health care reform requires accountable care systems. *JAMA* 2008;300:95–97.

3. Improving Health Care: A Dose of Competition: A Report by the Federal Trade Commission and the Department of Justice. July 2004. Available at <http://www.ftc.gov/ogc/healthcarehearings/index.htm> (accessed August 16, 2008).

4. Rosenthal MB. Payer model update. *N Engl J Med* 2008;359:1197–1200.

5. Medicare Payment Advisory Commission. Report to Congress: Reforming the Delivery System. June 2008. Available at <http://www.medpac.gov/documents/Jun08_EntireReport.pdf> (accessed August 16, 2008).

6. Hackbarth G, Reischauer R, Mutti A. Collective accountability for medical care: Toward bundled Medicare payments. *N Engl J Med* 2008;359:3–5.

7. Berwick DM, DeParle NA, Eddy DM, et al. Paying for performance: Medicare should lead. *Health Aff* November–December 2003;22:6:8–10.

8. Rosenthal MB, Landon BE, Normand ST, Frank RG, Ahmad TS, Epstein AE. Employers' use of value-based purchasing strategies. *JAMA* 2007;298:2281–2288.

9. Epstein AM. Pay for performance at the tipping point. *N Engl J Med* 2007;356:515–517.

10. Epstein AM, Lee TH, Hamel MB. Paying physicians for high-quality care. *N Engl J Med* 2004;350:406–410.

11. Rosenthal MB, Fernandopulle R, Song HR, Landon BE. Paying for quality: Providers' incentives for quality improvement. *Health Aff* 2004;23:127–141.

12. Rosenthal MB, Landon BE, Howitt K, Song HR, Epstein AM. Climbing up the pay-for-performance learning curve: Where are the early adopters now? *Health Aff* 2007;26:1674–1682.

13. Rosenthal MB, Dudley RA. Pay-for-performance: Will the latest payment trend improve care? *JAMA* 2007;297:740–743.

14. Hahn J. Pay-for-performance in health care. Congressional Research Service, Library of Congress, November 2, 2006. Available at <http://www.vascularweb.org/professionals/Government_Relations/PDF_Doc/CRS%20report%20on%20P4P.pdf> (accessed August 17, 2008).

15. Lindenauer PK, Remus D, Roman S, et al. Public reporting and pay for performance in hospital quality improvement. *N Engl J Med* 2007;356:486–496.

16. Kahneman D, Tversky A. Prospect theory: An analysis of decision under risk. *Econometrica* 1979;47:263–291.

17. Lee TH. Pay for performance, Version 2.0? *N Engl J Med* 2007;357:531–533.

18. Casale AS, Paulus RA, Selna MJ, et al. "ProvenCare™": A provider-driven pay-for-performance program for acute episodic cardiac surgical care. *Ann Surgery* 2007;245:613–623.

19. Miller HD. Creating Payment Systems to Accelerate Value-Driven Health Care: Issues and Options for Policy Reform. Commonwealth Fund, September 2007. Available at <http://www.commonwealthfund.org/publications/publications_show.htm?doc_id=522583> (accessed on August 16, 2008).

20. de Brantes F, Camillus JA. Evidence-Informed Case Rates: A New Health Care Payment Model. Commonwealth Fund, April 2007. Available at <http://www.commonwealthfund.org/publications/publications_show.htm?doc_id=478278> (accessed August 16, 2008).

21. Robinson JC, Casalino LP. Reevaluation of capitation contracting in New York and California. *Health Aff* Web exclusive, May 17, 2001. Available at <http://content.healthaffairs.org/cgi/content/full/hlthaff.w1.11v1/DC1?maxtoshow=&HITS=10&hits=10&RESULTFORMAT=&author1=Robinson&author2=Casalino&andorexacttitle=and&andorexacttitleabs=and&andorexactfulltext=and&searchid=1&FIRSTINDEX=0&sortspec_relevance&resourcetype=HWCIT> (accessed March 7, 2009).

22. Newhouse JP, Sinaiko AD. Can multi-payer financing achieve single-payer spending levels? *Forum for Health Economics and Policy* 2007;10:1:article 2. Available at <http://www.bepress.com/fhep/10/1/2> (accessed March 7, 2009).

Chapter 12: Market Change

1. Lee TH, Zapert K. Do high deductible health plans threaten quality of care? *N Engl J Med* 2005;353:1202–1204.

2. Reported in <http://www.ama-assn.org/amednews/2008/06/23/bil10623.htm> (accessed August 16, 2008).

3. Werner RM, Bradlow ET. Relationship between Medicare's Hospital Compare performance measures and mortality rates. *JAMA* 2006;296:2694–2702.

4. Pham HH, Coughlan J, O'Malley AS. The impact of quality-reporting programs on hospital operations. *Health Aff* 2006;25:1412–1422.

5. Dranove D, Kessler DP, McClellan M, Satterthwaite M. Is more information better? The effects of "report cards" on health care providers. *J Political Economy* 2003;111: 555–588.

6. Jha AK, Epstein AM. The predictive accuracy of the New York State coronary artery bypass surgery report-card system. *Health Aff* 2006;25:844–855.

7. Fung CH, et al. Systematic review: The evidence that publishing patient care performance data improves quality of care. *Ann Intern Med* 2008;148:111.

8. Werner RM, Asch DA. The unintended consequences of publicly reporting quality information. *JAMA* 2005;293:1239–1244.

9. Hibbard JH. What can we say about the impact of publish reporting? Inconsistent execution yields variable results. *Ann Intern Med* 2008;148:160.

10. Congressional Budget Office. Increasing Transparency in the Pricing of Health Care Services and Pharmaceuticals. June 5, 2008. Available at <http://www.cbo.gov/ftpdocs/92xx/doc9284/PriceTransparency.htm> (accessed July 14, 2008).

11. Parsons T. *The Social System.* New York: Free Press, 1964.

12. Fronstin P, Collins SR. The 2nd Annual EBRI/Commonwealth Fund Consumerisim in Health Care Survey, 2006: Early Experience with High-Deductible and Consumer-Driven Health Plans. EBRI Issue Brief No. 300, December 2006. Available at <http://www.ebri.org/publications/ib/index.cfm?fa=ibDisp&content_id=3769> (accessed March 7, 2009).

13. Available at <http://www.gao.gov/new.items/d08474r.pdf> (accessed July 16, 2008).

14. Buntin MB, Damberg C, Haviland A, et al. Consumer-directed health care: Early evidence about effects on cost and quality. *Health Aff* 2006;25:w516–w530.

15. Wharam JF, Landon BE, Galbraith AA, et al. Emergency department use and subsequent hospitalizations among members of a high-deductible health plan. *JAMA* 2007;297:1093–1102.

16. Wharam JF, Galbraith AA, Kleinman KP, Souerai SB, Ross-Degnan D, Landon BE. Cancer screening before and after switching to a high-deductible health plan. *Ann Intern Med* 2008;148:647–655.

17. Greene J, Hibbard J, Murray JF, Teutsch SM, Berger ML. The impact of consumer-directed health plans on prescription drug use. *Health Aff* 2008;27:1111–1119.

18. Rowe JW, Brown-Stevenson T, Downey RL, Newhouse JP. The effect of consumer-directed health plans on the use of preventive and chronic illness services. *Health Aff* 2008;27:113–120.

19. Christianson JB, Ginsburg PB, Draper DA. The transition from managed care to consumerism: A community level status report. *Health Aff* 2008;27:1362–1370.

Chapter 13: Accelerating Evolution

1. Porter ME, Teisberg EO. How physicians can change the future of health care. *JAMA* 2007;297:1103–1111.

2. Kahn R, Robertson RM, Smith R, Eddy D. The impact of prevention on reducing the burden of cardiovascular disease. *Circulation* 2008;118:576–585.

3. Cohen JT, Neumann PJ, Weinstein MC. Does preventive care save money? Health economics and the presidential candidates. *N Engl J Med* 2008;358:661–663.

4. Reinertsen JL. Zen and the art of autonomy maintenance. *Ann Intern Med* 2003; 138:993–995.

5. Jost TS, Emanuel EJ. Legal reforms necessary to promote delivery system innovation. *JAMA* 2008;299:2561–2563.

Further Readings

To develop the perspectives presented in this book, we drew on a wide range of books, articles from the peer-reviewed literature, and position papers and reports from foundations and government agencies. We will describe some resources that may be particularly useful for readers who want to go deeper in various areas.

There are numerous valuable reports from the Institute of Medicine, and the two that have been most influential in creating a consensus vision for the health care system that we need are *To Err Is Human: Building a Safer Health System* (2000) [1] and *Crossing the Quality Chasm: A New Health System for the 21st Century* (2001) [2]. The now-classic papers by Elizabeth McGlynn and colleagues [3, 4] that describe the frequency with which we fall short of this ideal are also essential reading for any student of health care delivery.

The Commonwealth Fund has taken a major leadership role in analyzing the performance of the U.S. health care system, and recommending strategies for its improvement. One of us (JJM) has had the privilege of chairing its Commission on a High Performance Health System, which has produced national and state-by-state scorecards in 2006 and 2008 [5, 6]. The Commonwealth Fund's Web site (<http://www.commonwealthfund.org/>) is a rich resource for any student of health care policy and provides access to numerous important papers that influenced this book [7–14].

Several thoughtful papers from government agencies and testimony by the leaders of these agencies are cited throughout this book. Of particular importance are the reports on health care issues from the CBO, which have addressed issues such as the role of technological progress in the growth of health care spending [15], the costs and benefits of health information technology [16], the impact and causes of geographic variation in health care spending [17], the potential value of comparative effectiveness evaluation as a strategy for reducing variation and mitigating the rate of rise of health care spending [18], and the impact of public reporting of prices of health care services and pharmaceuticals [19]. Another government agency, the Medicare Payment Advisory Commission, has helped define strategies for using payment methods to reform health care delivery [20].

Papers and books by Steve Shortell [21, 22], Larry Casalino [22, 23], and their colleagues have helped define the potential contribution of provider organization and care improvement systems. We cite only a few here, but their work on these topics has been influential over decades. Similarly, several papers by Meredith Rosenthal, Arnold Epstein, and their colleagues have provided an evolving assessment of pay-for-performance and other payment models [24–30].

We are far from being experts in behavioral economics and game theory, but have learned from and enjoyed books on topics including prospect theory [31], game theory [32], and negotiation strategies that are likely to lead most rapidly to cooperative relationships [33]. Our comments on system theory in chapter 10 drew on the work of the late father of one of the authors [34].

References

1. Committee on Quality of Health Care in America, Institute of Medicine. *To Err Is Human: Building a Safer Health System*. Washington, DC: National Academy Press, 2000.

2. Committee on Quality of Health Care in America, Institute of Medicine. *Crossing the Quality Chasm: A New Health System for the 21st Century*. Washington, DC: National Academy Press, 2001.

3. McGlynn EA, Asch SM, Adams J, et al. The quality of health care delivered to adults in the United States. *N Engl J Med* 2003;348:2635–2645.

4. Asch SM, Kerr EA, Keesey J, et al. Who is at greatest risk for receiving poor-quality health care? *N Engl J Med* 2006;354:1147–1156.

5. The Commonwealth Fund Commission on a High Performance Health System. Why Not the Best? Results from the National Scorecard on U.S. Health System Performance, September 2006. Available at <http://www.commonwealthfund.org/usr_doc/Commission_whynotthebest_951.pdf?section=4039> (accessed August 4, 2008).

6. The Commonwealth Fund Commission on a High Performance Health System. Why Not the Best? Results from the National Scorecard on U.S. Health System Performance, 2008. Available at <http://www.commonwealthfund.org/publications/publications_show.htm?doc_id=692682> (accessed July 29, 2008).

7. Zuckerman S, McFeeters J. Recent Growth in Health Expenditures. Commonwealth Fund, March 2006. Available at <http://www.cmwf.org/publications/publications_show.htm?doc_id=362803> (accessed February 18, 2007).

8. Davis K, Schoen C, Guterman S, Shih T, Schoenbaum SC, Weinbaum I. Slowing the Growth of U.S. Health Care Expenditures: What Are the Options? Commonwealth Fund, January 29, 2007. Available at <http://www.commonwealthfund.org/Content/Publications/Fund-Reports/2007/Jan/Slowing-the-Growth-of-U-S–Health-Care-Expenditures–What-Are-the-Options.aspx> (accessed March 7, 2009).

9. Commonwealth Fund Survey of Public Views of the U.S. Health Care System, 2008. Available at <http://www.commonwealthfund.org/surveys/surveys_show.htm?doc_id=698589> (accessed August 9, 2008).

10. 2002 Commonwealth Fund International Health Policy Survey. Available at <http://www.commonwealthfund.org/surveys/surveys_show.htm?doc_id=228168> (accessed August 9, 2008).

11. Miller HD. Creating payment systems to accelerate value-driven health care: Issues and options for policy reform. Commonwealth Fund, September 2007. Available at <http://www.commonwealthfund.org/publications/publications_show.htm?doc_id=522583> (accessed August 16, 2008).

12. de Brantes F, Camillus JA. Evidence-informed case rates: A new health care payment model. Commonwealth Fund, April 2007. Available at <http://www.commonwealthfund.org/publications/publications_show.htm?doc_id=478278> (accessed August 16, 2008).

13. Beal AC, Doty MM, Hernandez SE, Shea KK, Davis K. Closing the Divide. Commonwealth Fund 2006 Health Care Quality Survey. Available at <http://www.commonwealthfund.org/surveys/surveys_show.htm?doc_id=506847> (accessed August 10, 2008).

14. Davis K, Schoenbaum SC, Audet AJ. A 2020 Vision of Patient-Centered Primary Care. Commonwealth Fund. Available at <http://www.commonwealthfund.org/usr_doc/868_Davis_2020_patient-centered_care_JGIM_10–2005_.pdf?section=4039> (accessed August 10, 2008).

15. Congressional Budget Office. Technological Change and the Growth of Health Care Spending. January 2008. Available at <http://www.cbo.gov/ftpdocs/89xx/doc8947/01–31–TechHealth.pdf> (accessed July 30, 2008).

16. Congressional Budget Office. Evidence on the Costs and Benefits of Health Information Technology. May 2008. Available at <http://www.cbo.gov/ftpdocs/95xx/doc9572/07–24–HealthIT.pdf> (accessed August 7, 2008).

17. Congressional Budget Office. Geographic Variation in Health Care Spending, February 2008. Available at <http://www.cbo.gov> (accessed August 12, 2008).

18. Congressional Budget Office. Research on the Comparative Effectiveness of Medical Treatments: Issues and Options for an Expanded Federal Role. December 2007 Available at <http://www.cbo.gov> (accessed August 12, 2008).

19. Congressional Budget Office. Increasing Transparency in the Pricing of Health Care Services and Pharmaceuticals, June 5, 2008. Available at <http://www.cbo.gov/ftpdocs/92xx/doc9284/PriceTransparency.htm> (accessed July 14, 2008).

20. Medicare Payment Advisory Commission. Report to Congress: Reforming the Delivery System. June 2008. Available at <http://www.medpac.gov/documents/Jun08_EntireReport.pdf> (accessed August 16, 2008).

21. Shortell SM, Gillies RR, Anderson DA, Erickson KM, Mitchell JB. *Remaking Health Care in America: The Evolution of Organized Delivery Systems.* 2nd ed. San Francisco: Jossey-Bass, 2000.

22. Shortell SM, Casalino LP. Health care reform requires accountable care systems. *JAMA* 2008;300:95–97.

23. Casalino LP. Disease management and the organization of physician practice. *JAMA* 2005;293:485–488.

24. Rosenthal MB, Landon BE, Normand ST, Frank RG, Ahmad TS, Epstein AE. Employers' use of value-based purchasing strategies. *JAMA* 2007;298:2281–2288.

25. Rosenthal MB. Beyond pay-for-performance: Emerging models of provider-payment reform. *N Engl J Med* 2008;359:1197–1200.

26. Epstein AM. Pay for performance at the tipping point. *N Engl J Med* 2007;356:515–517.

27. Epstein AM, Lee TH, Hamel MB. Paying physicians for high-quality care. *N Engl J Med* 2004;350:406–410.

28. Rosenthal MB, Fernandopulle R, Song HR, Landon BE. Paying for quality: Providers' incentives for quality improvement. *Health Aff* 2004;23:127–141.

29. Rosenthal MB, Landon BE, Howitt K, Song HR, Epstein AM. Climbing up the pay-for-performance learning curve: Where are the early adopters now? *Health Aff* 2007;26:1674–1682.

30. Rosenthal MB, Dudley RA. Pay-for-performance: Will the latest payment trend improve care? *JAMA* 2007;297:740–743.

31. Kahneman D, Tversky A. *Choices, Values, and Frames.* Cambridge: Cambridge University Press, 2000.

32. Poundstone W. *Prisoner's Dilemma.* New York: Doubleday, 1992.

33. Axelrod R. *The Evolution of Cooperation.* New York: Basic Books, 1985.

34. Lee TH, Shiba S, Wood RC. *Integrated Management Systems: A Practical Approach to Transforming Organizations.* New York: Wiley, 1999.

Index